B U T T E R F L Y R A M M Y

BUTTERFLY RAMMY

THE ART OF SCOTLAND'S POLITICAL AWAKENING

Published by Common Print
August 2015
ISBN 978-0-9930965-2-5

Printed and bound in Great Britain
by Thomson the Printers,
14 Carnoustie Place,
Glasgow G5 8PB

COMMON PRINT

Common Print is the publishing arm
of the Common Weal

allofusfirst.org

Index

The Project

On September 18 2014 Scotland was asked to vote on whether or not it wanted to become an independent country. The campaign for a Yes vote stimulated a wide, diverse grassroots campaign that involved many creative voices in a discussion of what Scotland is and could be. Despite the No vote, this movement has created a political awakening in Scotland that has entirely changed the nature of our national debate. Common Weal is a think and do tank whose ideas about a fairer, more equal society played a major role during the campaign.

To mark the year since the last days of that campaign it has commissioned 18 artists and 18 writers to reflect on what happened, following the arc of events through 18 Scots words which capture the their spirit. These formed the basis of a month of cabarets at the Edinburgh Festival - and this book.

Author and artist information is available from the Butterfly Rammy webpage.

Prints of the artworks are available for purchase.

All quotations are credited on page 112.

allofusfirst.org/rammy

commonspace.scot

Prologue
Robin McAlpine

What a strange and disorientating thing, to awake from a dwam. When the cotton wool haze of a meandering daydream leaves us, when our mind comes back from elsewhere, when our concentration returns to us the sharpness of our surroundings. Falling out from a dwam you will find the cold suddenly colder, the warmth warmer. For how long have you been here?

So how long was it? Perhaps since the doors opened again on a Parliament for Scotland. It was such a long road to those doors that as they swung apart before us did we perhaps mistake its threshold for a destination? In that dwam, in that place, did we perhaps coo 'it'll do, it'll do'. A bit better. Not quite as bad. Let's shop.

It'll do. It'll do.

Naw it wilny.

And it won't because someone asks us the question "Do you want Scotland to be an independent country?". A cotton wool haze begins to lift, our surroundings sharper again, the cold colder, the warmth warmer. Do we? Do we?

As our senses return, we feel the drooth, the thirst for something. Is it a thirst for our independence? Not sure – but it's definitely a drooth. Not just this, surely? Something more, surely? And yet it all begins so dour. Her spreadsheet. His spreadsheet. Who wins? Do I care? At first, he says 'it's No for the same', but then she says 'it's Yes for the same – mostly'.

Ah, we Scots have a way with dull greys. Look at our cooncil hooses. On a bad day they match the sky. But how, how can this question be a dull grey?

It'll do.

Naw it wilny.

So we get to gabbin. No-one came with a 'conversation' neatly folded in the boot of their leased, silver, is-it-not-too-big-for-one-person car. Just us. Talking. All at once. Over the top of each other. A new sentence before the old one is finished. It didn't feel grey. It's wasn't. This was no longer Kansas.

And so to that other thing the Scots do so well – shall we call it wild? Certainly untamed. First day of summer with no rain and it's straight in the river for a dook. No, of course you can't feel your legs. First real snow of the winter and men in business suits are chucking snowballs at each other. And yes it looks strange. Steal a kiss off a bemused Estonian police woman at the football, climb a statue and put a traffic cone on its head, get asked by a tourist where to get lunch and walk them half a mile to the best chippy in town.

It'll no last. Better make the most of it.

That's what happened. No-one handed us the campaign we wanted (like no-one has handed us the country we wanted). So what is there to be done? Dour or untamed? Fuck it, sun's oot, taps aff. We'll just need to make our own.

But where? And how? And what if no-one comes? This isn't a construction project. No-one is wearing hard hats and there's no budget.

It's your gran, the guy that works in the bank, your hairdresser. And then (no-one is more surprised by this than you) – it's you. You'll just need to build it from whatever you have and keep it wherever you can.

What about the toon hall? Did they not use to use them for this sort of stuff? That guy, I liked what he said yon time. That woman – do you think she'd come? Will we ask them? Let's ask them. So-and-so could knock up some posters and some leaflets if so-and-so could sneak-photocopy them at her work. But I can only play the fiddle? Fine, play the fiddle. Folk'll like it.

If they come. What if they dinnae come? Ma nails are bit tae pieces. Hold on, here's someone. And here's someone else. And someone else. Jesus – have you seen it in there? It's hoachin. Actual hoachin.

The following morning a young man thinks about the meeting. He went in curious but a bit embarrassed (folk don't do this kind of thing, what am I doing here?), head down like he was auditing the lines of the badminton court. He came out different. The thing that he thought he thought, mibby he doesn't think it after all. Why did he think it? Can he remember why he thought it? This is strange. Why is he asking himself questions? Might it be less strange to write it down? He writes it down. He puts it on his Facebook. And then – holy fuck! – five thousand people read it. Some of them send links to answer his questions. He discovers Bella, Wings, Wee Ginger Dug, National Collective, Radical Indy. He reads and learns and reads and learns. Stuff he never thought he'd read. Stuff he never thought he'd learn. See when ye ken stuff, there's nae cause fir being embarrassed. When he walks into his local Yes hub his head isn't down. Is there anything he can do?

None of this is big. It's tiny. Lots and lots of tiny. None of this is grey. It's bright. It's flashes of sunlight all over the place. It becomes kind of mesmerising. It doesn't look like a thing. It doesn't stand, it swirls. Can you see some kind of order in this? I can't. It looks like chaos, like a rammy in the pub. But it's not violent. So small, so delicate, so colourful.

A butterfly rammy? Aye, a butterfly rammy.

Is the question 'Where do you bide?'. Is this about here, about being from here? Of course it is. And of course it's not. We'd all like to fix everywhere – but how are we going to do that if we don't fix here? Where we bide. Does mending your own roof mean you wish other people were wet? How does us being wet too help? Is 'here' a reason? Mibby aye, mibby naw – but it's not the only one. So some of us carry flags and some of us don't. One thing we all are is scunnered. Sick to the back teeth of someone trying to put us back into our dwam. We've felt cold colder and it'll no do. Not at all. Hope and anger? Those we all carry.

Someone outside notices that it's not just the yellows, that it's the greens and the reds too. But why can't they see the mauves, lilacs, tangerines, turquoises, maroons, azures, cerises and indigos? They keep assuming that a tangerine must be a yellow in disguise, that a turquoise is the same thing as a green. They're wrong. We're shades, not categories. We're lots and lots of things. We're friends now. We don't greet each other in concepts but with hugs. The more they call us fake yellow, the happier we become in our rainbow. We coorie doon thigither. Many of us will remember this with more happiness than you will believe.

Others are beelin. Ragin. Very angry indeed. We live here too, they say. Why are you trying to take away our here? Why are you trying to make us live in your here? Oddly, the more they have, the angrier they are. But this really is their here too. Mibby we could talk?

No you can't. Wheesht. We're the fucking news and we'll decide who talks. Wheesht. We're the fucking news and we'll decide what you hear, who's good, who's bad, what numbers are real numbers and what numbers are not real numbers. Oh, by the way, you'll be hearing no noises of hope. You're the bad guys and your numbers are not real numbers.

And so a nation swithers. On the one hand this. On the other hand that. And then, nearly at the end, one moment when it looks like it could be the left hand. And so, from London, come banks and supermarkets and mobile phone companies and the Daily Record, united in their goal of cutting that hand right off. No money, no food, no phones. Do as you're told and we'll give you magic beans. Well, actually, a vow. (Can't we have the magic beans instead? No? But what the fuck can we do with a vow?)

A blur. A great big flurry of exhausted butterflies. Is that us really here? A blur. A blur.

And then it's a driech morning. Weeks of sun and the grey is back. It's like the weather knew.

No.

It rains.

Were we just too feart? Was that all it was? Did we live in a here that was too small, not big enough to fit those who lived in that other here? Was it us? Was it them? We'd be angry if we could stop crying. Numb. Today the cold doesn't feel cold and the warm doesn't feel warm. Is that it? Are the butterflies gone for good? Now I'm feart.

But that carpet of lifeless butterflies twitches. The most amazing thing. No-one asks us, no-one tells us. But we find ourselves back in the square again. Leaving food for the poor. Thousands of us. Our here is still here. We're still here. The young man blogs, the hairdresser volunteers, the granny joins, the guy from the bank donates. What are we doing? Anything, just anything. This isn't over. Thrawn? Aye we're thrawn. Did you think we were kidding? This isn't over.

What a strange and disorientating thing, to know that everything has changed. To know it was us. To know we're still here.

Mind. Mind how it felt. Mind who we were. Mind what we did. Mind why we did it. They want us to forget. They want everyone to forget. You weren't that nation. You weren't those people. Sleep children sleep. And we'll coo 'it'll do, it'll do'.

Naw. It. Fucking. Wilny.

Mind.

Dwam

A reverie, a trivial daydream, losing connection with reality.

Scotland had a lower turnout rate in elections than the rest of the UK. It was not a nation of activists. After a period of Westminster politics dominated by the mantra of 'There is no alternative', Scotland was as if in a daydream, shopping and watching the football. Then we woke up.

Has Britain been in a dwam?
How did Scotland wake up?

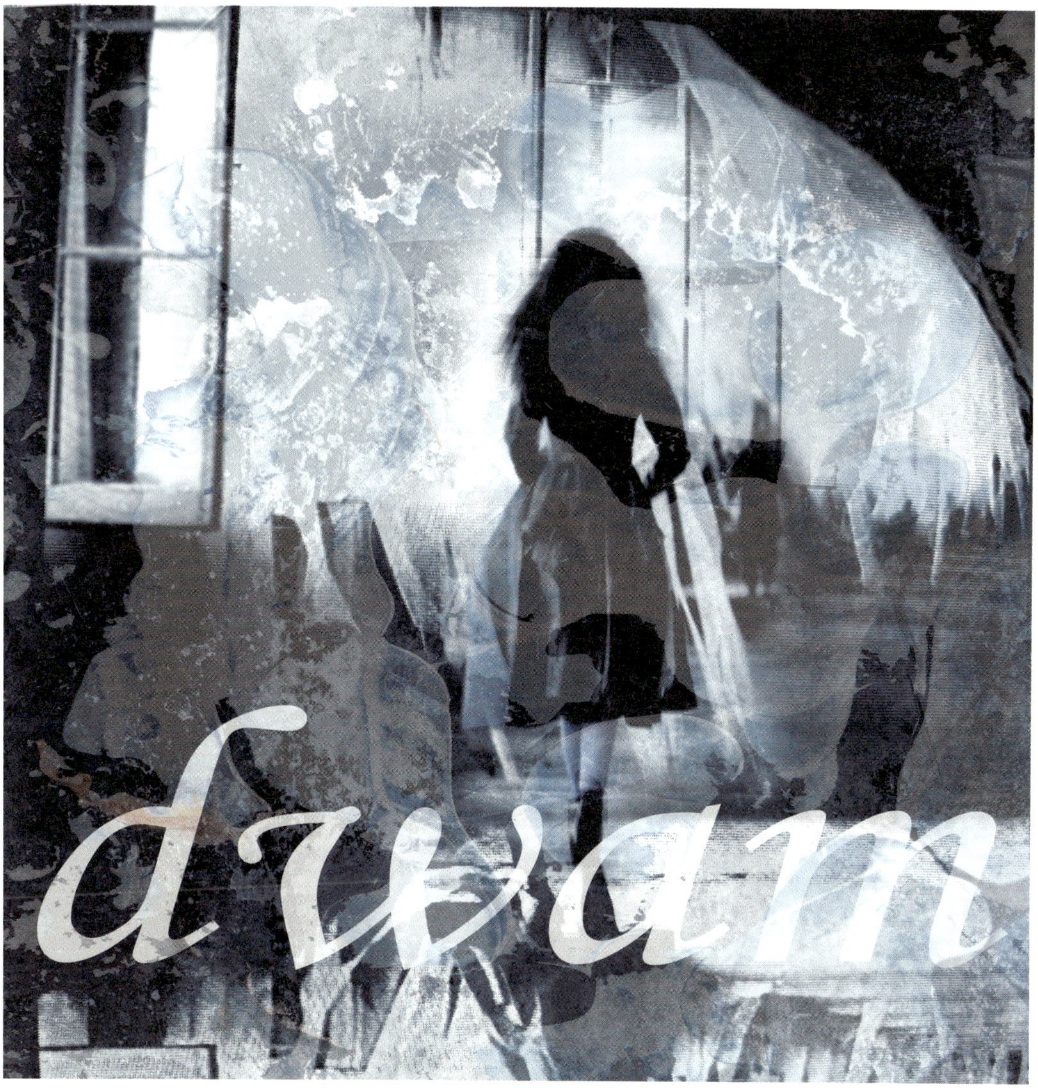

Dwam
Elspeth Lamb

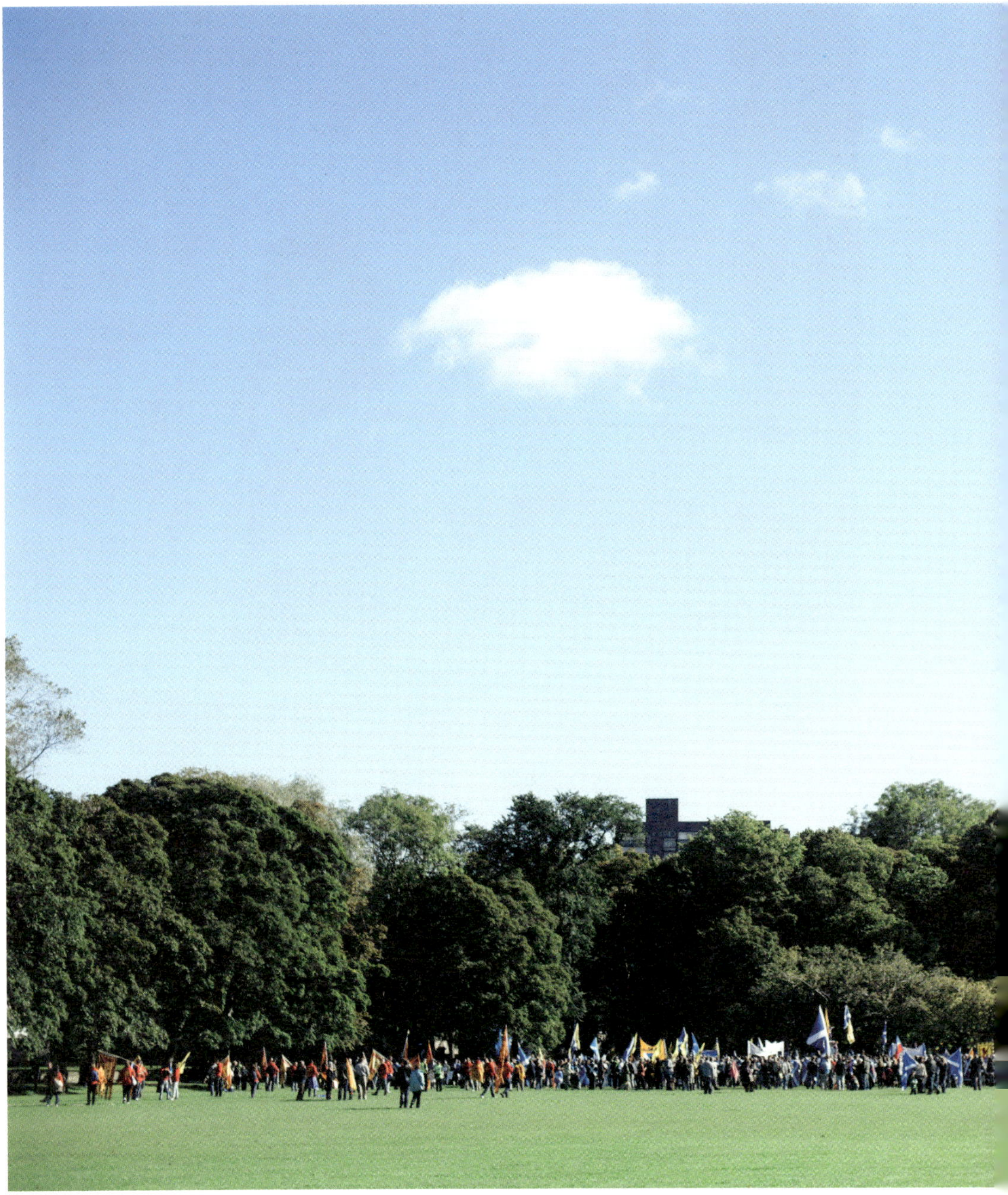

"For some of the young group, voting was treated almost with disdain: if you voted then you were being manipulated. 'Do you think I'm zipped up the back?' was a response from one member of this group when asked about voting. 'I'm no giving any of them my vote' also implied a sense that their vote was valuable and important, but none of the options on offer were worthy of it. Significantly, participants tended not to discriminate between different types of election when discussing their reasons for not voting. This reflected a deep level of distrust in politicians, as well as participants' general lack of confidence that their vote would make a difference."

Willie Sullivan

Extract from *The Missing Scotland: Why over a million Scots choose not to vote and what it means for our democracy*

Dwam
Karen Campbell

You tried to tell her what a dwam was.

'You mean like whisky?' Mocking the word, so the w toe-curls a la Elmer Fudd. 'Aye, I like a drwam.' Opening the shutters, which are green.

So you talk about swimming, that time on holiday when the loch was freezing in the vivid sun, how you close your eyes and plunge in, and there's the rhythm and the rhythm, how the bright blue breaks above you, but you are under it, and warm, how the rhythm and the rhythm it is warm and monotonous and you just get on with it, although you know the bright blue breaks above you.

'I don't like to get my hair wet,' she says as she splashes cold water on her face.

So you talk about the tousled morning, when you half-wake and you stretch out your limbs, to feel the extremities your extremities can reach and it is further than the furthest thing, because the sheets and the breaking day are infinite, then. 'You know?' you say.

'I hate long lies,' she says as she pours the porridge.

So you take her on a walk, and your arms are swinging, your hand in hers, you make it swing. And there is no talking, just the rhythm, the monotonous, meditative rhythm which is your closeness, how you used to always see the same things, and you take her past the furthest outskirts of your run-down town. Past the empty poverty to the yawning hills. The Faerie Hill.

'That's us,' you laugh, and you wait for her to say it. But she doesn't, so you do. 'Away with the fairies.'

But she doesn't smile. So you try to explain, how there's a stupor about it, a sense of self-induced thrawnness that is deeper than a dream, how it shimmers, how the reality shimmers round about and you can see it, there, outside of your bubble, but you can tell yourself it's not real.

'It's like it's easier,' you say. 'But it's not.'

She says she's cold, so you walk back home, and the rhythms of your feet are jarring. So you talk about that film, The Matrix, which she likes, seeing as Keanu's in a leather coat throughout. About how a cat's cradle can rock you blind, and it's a nice swing, at first, if you let it be, but when you see the actual cat gut, how it crisses and crosses and cuts into your flesh, then the rhythm can make you seasick.

'I wouldny go on a boat,' she says. 'Not a wee one anyway. You know me. Claustrophobic.'

So you talk about climbing out of it, the safe, rocking dark. How you blink at first, how you see a lot of bad stuff, crap stuff, like the slaters on the underside of a stone. You tell her how you find things that were always right can be wrong .

'Like you?' she says, as she cooks the kale. 'You wanting ham with your dwam?'

'Naw. Just Spam,' you say.

And she laughs, and pours you a drink.

So you sip your drink, and she sips hers, and you try to tell her about the mellowness, how nice and quiet that is. How your dad gave you your first taste of beer. How you miss being wee and have folk doing stuff for you, miss the summery waste of time when you built your dens and just came in for tea.

'Me too,' she says, as she does the dishes.

You open more cans and you talk about hangovers, how they're shit, all that waking up with a carpet on your tongue, and the grey shaking day looms and you just go back to bed.

'Mind and make that your last then.' She flicks you with the dishcloth, which you catch, and pull her close. You hook your finger through her vest strap. You love her in vest tops, the way they uphold the finest of her fine curves. That dip where the muscle of her arm is flexed.

'It is like the cold,' you say. 'The way it shocked you. You know. That time in the loch. But remember when we came out afterwards? How alive we felt?'

She shivers.

You talk about how the water widened your eyes, so the world was sharp and open. How you'd noticed that other path between the trees, the longer, broader one, and all the new paths branching wide.

'Aye, and we got lost twice,' she says, as she reaches to close the shutters.

You catch her wrist. Not hard. 'But we did it,' you say.

'And I missed EastEnders.' She ruffles your hair. 'See you. You'll be wanting to do orienteering next.'

'Let's have a toast.'

She rolls her eyes.

'To us,' you say. 'To Scotland.' And you are in that dwam, where the warmth and the brightness bulks you up, you knock your glass and it spills, oblique, pouring out all the hidden sport and sunshine, the passion and debate, the talking, the knowing, the pride. How you can't unknow what you know now. How you can't unsee the dreams you saw, and how the mirror showed who you might be.

'I'm proud,' you say.

'You're pished.' She takes your glass away.

So you speak again of reverie. You tell her that there's imminence in the air; how it rises yet. How you don't want to pass the baton, you want to share it.

'Please,' you say. 'I'll just wait here. You catch me up.'

You stand there in your jammies and you cast out a thread, a line of catgut maybe, or a silver filament of self-esteem, you don't know anymore because you're in your dwam and you're in your cups and she's nursing her wrath to keep it warm.

You tried to tell her, what a dwam was. She saw it as a slap.

'You calling me stupid?' she said. 'Come to bed.'

Drooth

A thirst most often affecting those in the days after excessive inebriation. See also: bevvy, swally, ginger.

Decades of managerial politics created a Britain where ideas, vision and inspiration were thin on the ground. When Scotland awoke during the referendum campaign, it was immediately noticed just how thirsty for ideas we all were.

Why has Britain lost a progressive vision of its future? How did Scotland find one?

"Scotland wills itself to be a better nation, one we rebuild with our own hands.

Who then will tell us our will is not big enough?

Who then will tell us our hands are not strong enough?"

RIC declaration 2013

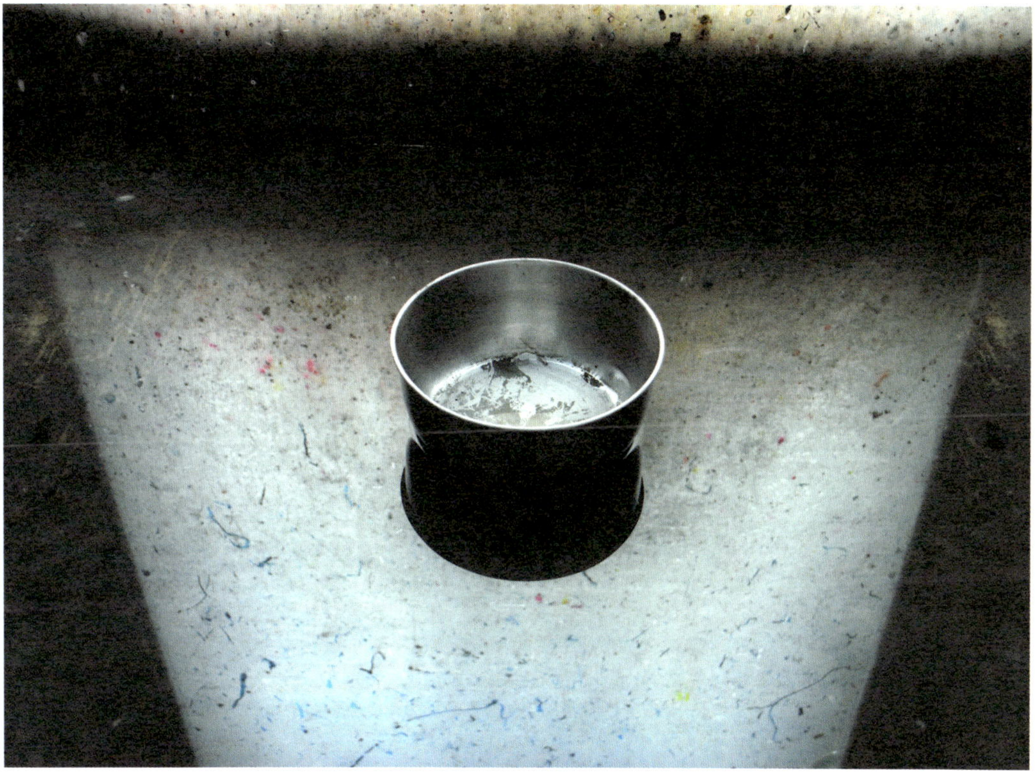

Drooth
Claire Forsyth

The Back o the Ha

Stuart McHardy

The cry came up as usual
fae near the back o the ha
the place whaur the puir fowk hunker
that bide tween the win an the wa
'Whit is this we ye crack o,
as yer wards grease the bools in yer mooth?
ye've nivver felt hungerin's slaver
this 'we' kens naethin o drooth,
thon terrible drooth fer freedom
tae hae things the wey we wuid like
wi'oot yer poleetical con-gemmes
that only suroond us wi dikes,
there ta mak siccar that preevilige
bides jist as it is fer the few
an them that accept ye as leaders
jist bigg up their prisons anew.

But as ye gie yer aw fer the nation
ye're jist ike the rest o yer ilk
peyin fer yer bairns' eddication
dressin yer douce wives in silk.
An then ye come back an ye tell us
we're aw o us on the same side
but we ken whit ye're tryin tae sell us
an we ken hou aften ye've tried
an ivver ye mind us o freedom
but yer freedom's jist no warth a toss
fer we're nou a wee bittie canny
sae think politics is jist a cross
scrievit on a wee bittie paper
ivvery five years or so
that yer cub cin continue tae function
an yer influence continue tae grow.

An ye come back an tell us we're British
an remind us o aw ye hae duin
but as soon as the coontin is ower
we ken fine whaur it is ye will run;
back tae the Bigtoon like lightnin
tae strut an tae pose mang yer freens
siccar ye've maistert the recknin
o pouer, o wealth an o dreams
an back here we're aince mair forgotten
like a backyaird fair throttlit wi weeds
oor pronle's nae warth takkin tent o
an mickle concern fer oor needs,
then ye fill up oor laun wi corruption
wasteland, pollution an bombs
an ainc mair our touns ken starvation
an aince mair the rickets returns.

Weel, we ken weel that this is yer midden
whaur aw things unsichtly are hid
but thistles aye best grow unbidden
lang eftir it's thocht they are died
so ye cin tak yer fine wards an orations
an keep pleyin at yer auld gemmes
ilk day ther's mair ken yer fictions
created in guid freedom's name
an we ken fine whit it is ye are daein
claimin tae wark fer us aw
cin ye no hear the chain-links snappin
up here at the back o the ha?

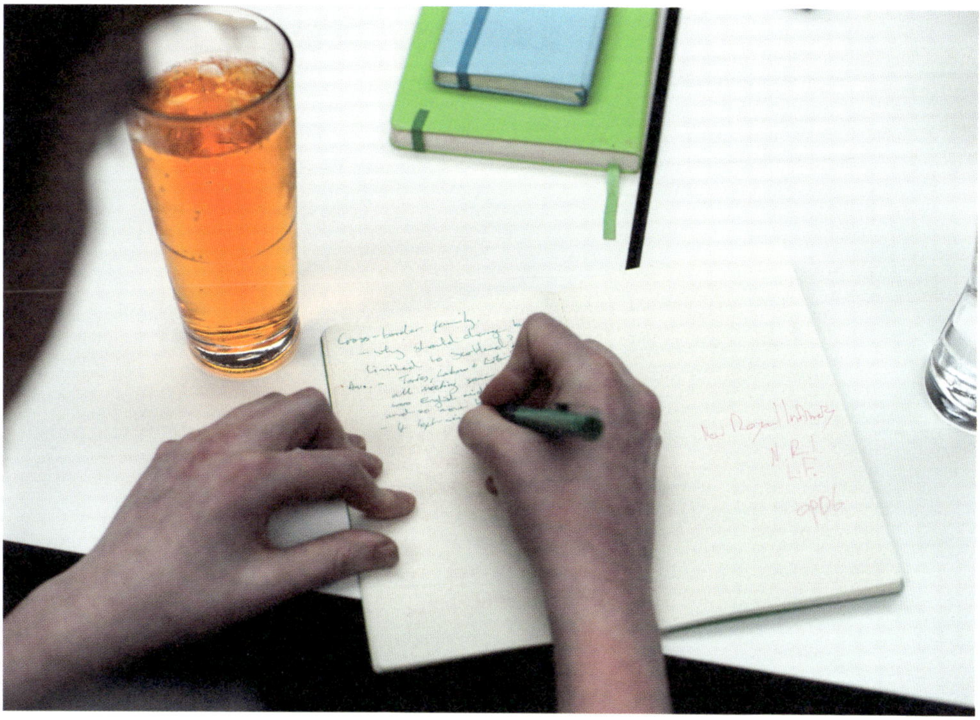

Peter McNally / Documenting Yes

Dour

A sullen and surly disposition, often observed as a face which trips oneself as it is so long. See also: Crabbit.

The earliest phases of the referendum campaign were uninspiring and focussed on technical issues. It seemed like the conversation was dominated by topics only of interest to accountants. This was turned around by the grassroots of the campaign which contextualised the vote for ordinary people.

When did politics become little more than elaborate bookkeeping? Why are political parties of all types so afraid of inspiring?

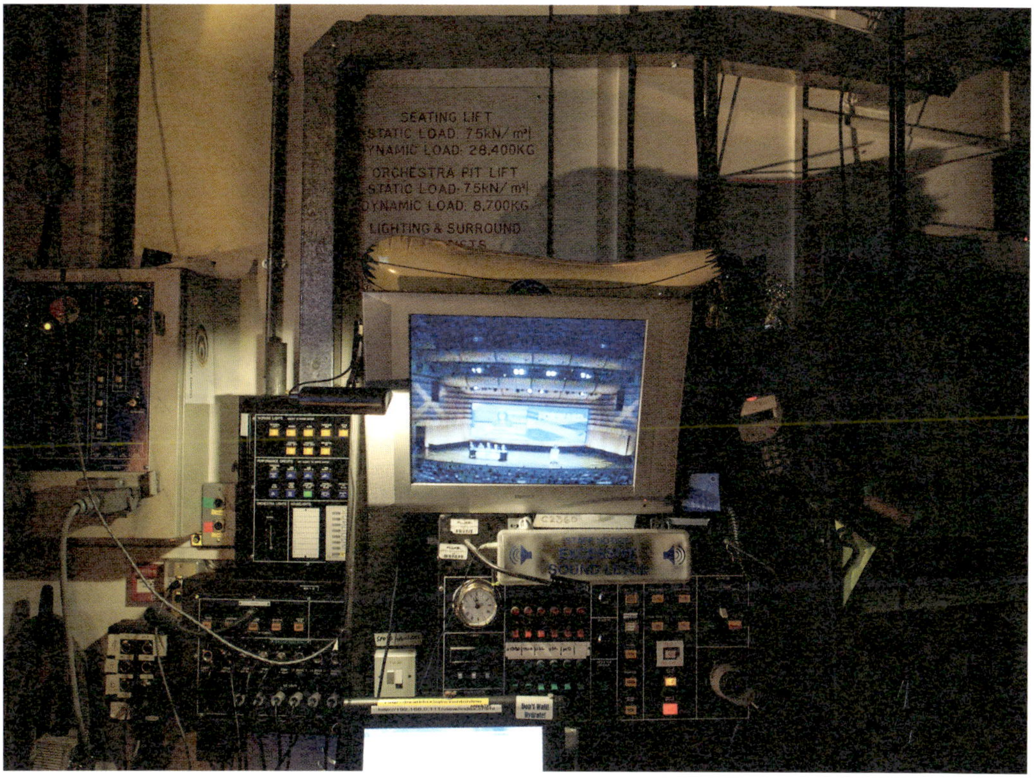
SEATING LIFT
ORCHESTRA PIT LIFT
LIGHTING & SURROUND

Dour

Gav Prentice

Let me tell you what you are. I have two stories for you at once. You're dour. You're not really dour enough.

Dourness is an intrinsic characteristic of Scottishness, hand in hand with being spendthrift sensibles that keep the heed. You are basically miserable tight-arses.

You are also the opposite of this. The Conservatives are left with the grim task of getting the books back in order and overly emotional Scots, the drunk-on-hope (or just drunk) subsidy junkies (or just junkies) that you are, can't understand that. You spend like Greeks, and let your brave hearts rule your judgement when you should be looking at the hard facts beyond hard noses.

Both of these stories are true at once.

Your culture is dour. You are a nation of entertainers.

Your music is particularly dour, your national anthem, now that's one of the clearest examples of dourness you could ever find. Let's mourn our nationality with a dirge eh? (I quite like it by the way.) Your football team's dour, they walk out that tunnel like somebody just showed them a dead puppy in the dressing room, they stand listening to said dirge for a minute, faintly mouthing away something or other, then following the on-pitch failure The Greatest Supporters On Earth cheer and applaud like it was a victory. So you even your celebration is dour. You know you'll take the high road and get there before me because you'll be dead, right?

Your language is dour. All of those Germanic noises interspersing English words just to make them angrier, you know how it makes you sound.

You sound like you're ready to shout "Freedom!" at any minute. You are the nation of Mel Gibson with a painted face, and you are also, at the same time, the nation of Adam Smith, soberly telling the industrialised world in painstaking detail how it was already operating and explaining why it should carry on as it was. If Adam Smith had a battle cry, which he never would, it would be that thus far, philosophers have changed the world in various ways, and the point is to interpret it.

Thatcher loved him. And you hate her. Before her though, there was a time when real conservatism was huge in Scotland. That's still who you are, really.

You are Nationalist Socialists. That is who you are, really. These are just the facts, and you cannot escape your destiny.

The last Scottish Prime Minister was the dourest Scotsman of all dour Scotsmen, he was the Platonic Form of dour, the child of the manse turned iron chancellor, always wittering on about economic growth. He was a classic Scottish tight-arse. He was also the opposite of that. He sold off all of the gold and got us into all of the debt. He spent like a lottery winner from the high flats, and never once forced a successful replication of a smile in the process. He was truly both stories at once. These are the facts. He was "a Socialist Scot who wants to spend every penny you earn. Never forget that." **(Kelvin MacKenzie)**

All of those Labour cabinets dominated by Scots with an upside-down smile lipsticked onto their pitbull faces. All of those John Reid TV appearances, seething, chippie, and overwhelmingly dour. All of those Labour MPs, for so long. All of those union leaders. All of that bevvy. All of that masochistic victimhood. A conservative country deep down. "I mean, down here we live under a sort of Scottish Raj." **(Jeremy Paxman)**

You are the nation of Mags Hainey routing the peadophiles. You are the nation of Gordon Brown during those No campaign speeches: "British Workers of British Work, unite! You have nothing to lose but your pensions!"

You don't spend money in shops, not real money, you expect the state to do your spending for you. You can measure that, it has been measured. You don't spend enough. Numbers are numbers and economic fact is economic fact, and those things are truisms. Facts like that if there is no third runway at Gatwick the economy of your capital city will collapse. Facts like that the recovery does not require a third runway at Gatwick and blue is the new green. Facts like that Greeks are not productive. Facts like that Greeks work more hours per week than we do. Facts like that if Scotland had come through for Labour in the end we wouldn't be facing a Tory budget. Facts like that if every man, woman and child in Scotland could and did vote Labour we would be facing exactly the same budget. Facts like that Scotland is still Labour deep down. Facts like that Scotland is as conservative a country as anywhere else.

These are the stories about who you are, and they have been told, from within and without, for a lot longer than the last three years. So that's what you are. Both of these. Evidence notwithstanding.

What interests me, is not whether Scotland will be automatically, certainly, admitted to various trans-national alliances. It's that we appear, as a nation, to place the utmost value on inter-dependence and international community, not just tactically, or in pursuit of trade, but existentially, and as a matter of principle.

Karine Polwart

Extract from *Imagination Vital to Telling the Yes Story*

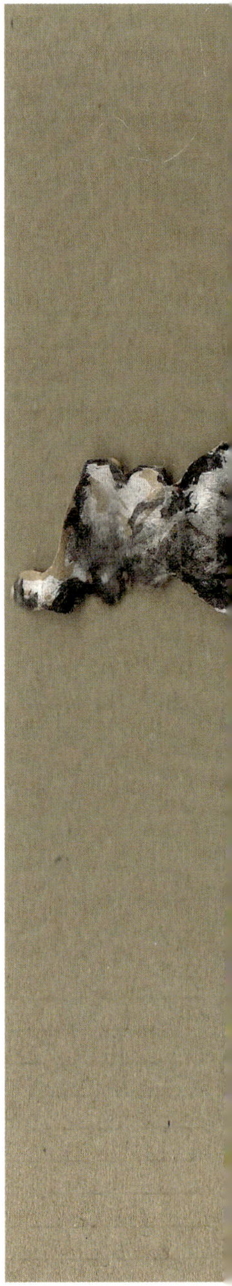

Dour
Charlotte Duffy AKA Waste of Paint Productions

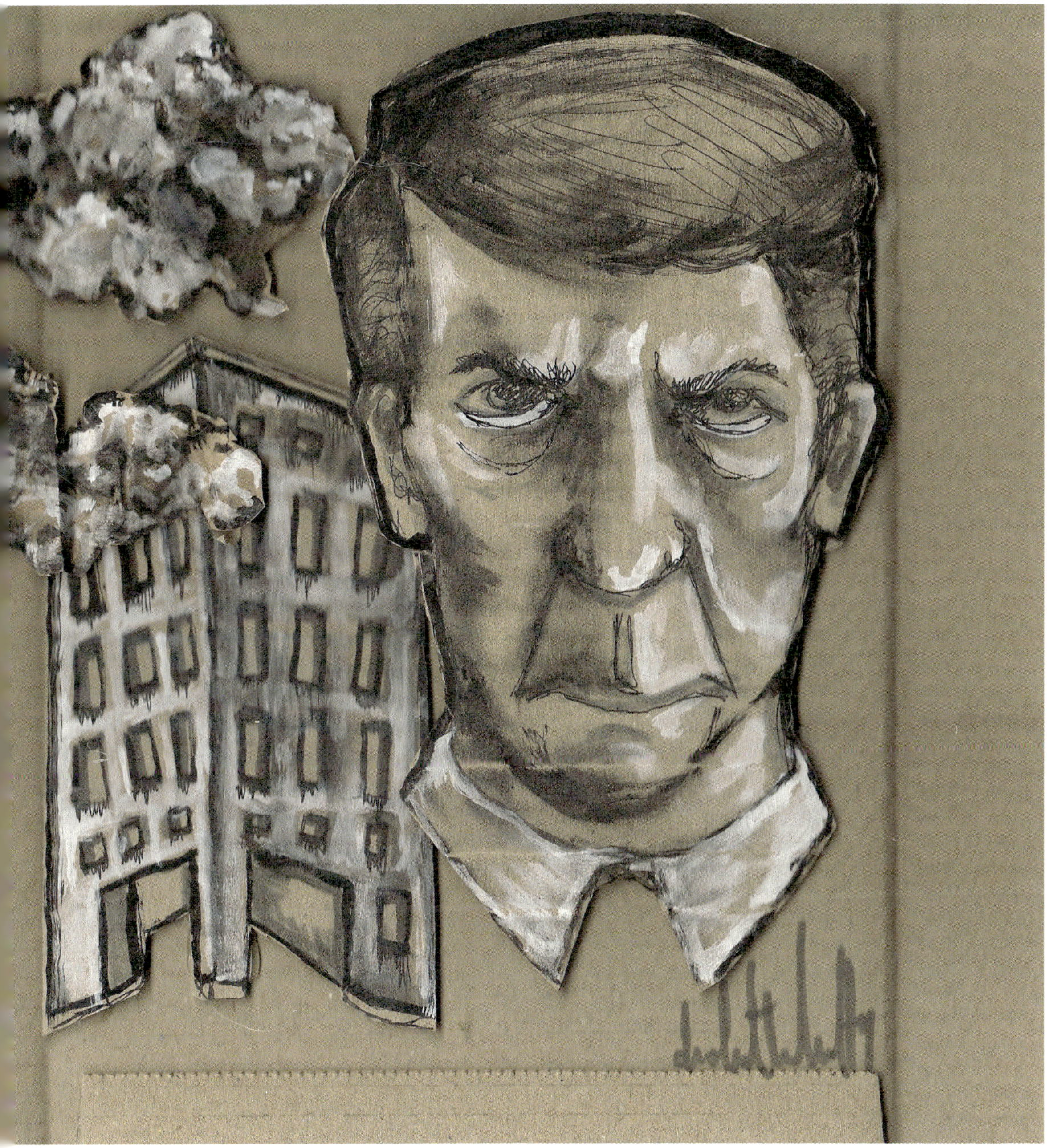

Gabbin (v)

Enthusiastic communication
between acquaintances.
"I went doon the shops to get the messages and spent an hour gabbin wae our Morag".

In the absence of an inspiring debate in the media, the grassroots of the independence campaign started to talk amongst themselves, expanding debates, imagining futures, and engaging more and more people in the conversation —and they liked what they heard.

Has politics become more cautious than its electorate? Is public activism the solution?

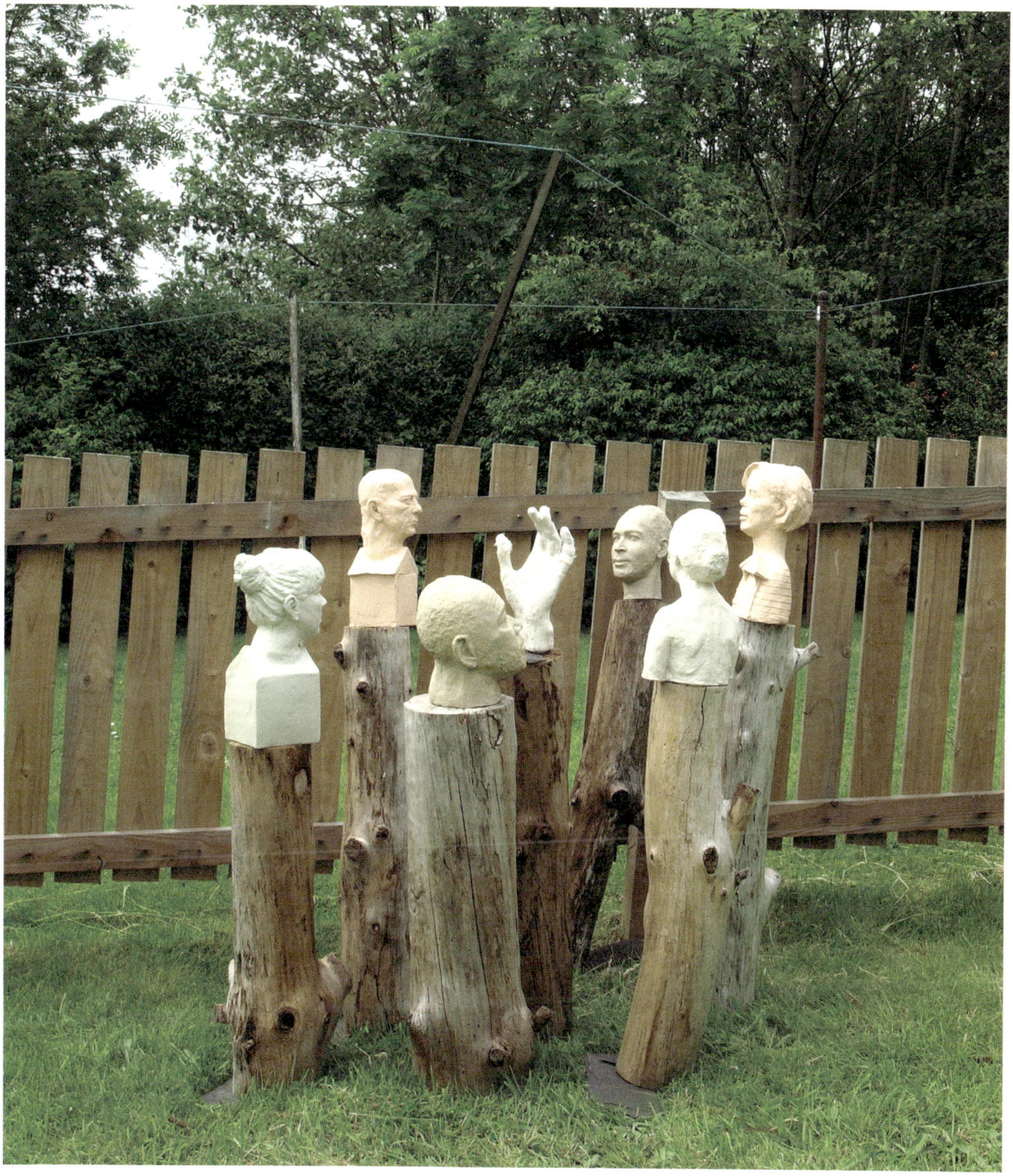

Gabbin
Nicola Carberry

Teach me

Agnes Török

Teach me how to be an ally to your struggle
tell me how to be strong for the both of us
when I am beat
when I am beat down and bloodied
when newspaper articles and election results
have pushed my heart deep underground
frozen for winter
not to thaw until a new kind of arab spring springs
from all that is broken about this world
when I feel hopeless and lost
when I give in and I give up
hand me something to fight with
that doesn't involve throwing rocks
give me something to fight *for*
that doesn't include hating those who fight *against*

don't let me be a **them**
to your battle
instead
tell me your stories
sing me your struggle songs
and I will do the same for you

teach me how to be an ally to your struggle
I am good listener
I make decent coffee for political meeting
and hospital waiting rooms
and I can hold hands as well as I can hold placards
so sit down next to me
and let's talk
let's talk

like it matters
because it does
because it is one of few things that always does
            count
this figuring out how to live together thing
this figuring out how to live with ourselves

In a world of political promises as hollow as bones
it is easy to train fists before training arguments
in a world of paper manifestos
it is easy to burn too bright
for due process
in a system **this flammable**
it is not strange
some of us would rather start the fire
than build futures
if we still have to watch them burn

So teach me how to be an ally
to your struggle
because I need to do something that matters
something that creates and innovates
something that restarts my sense of purpose
beyond myself

teach me how to be an ally to your struggle
because I cannot live happily alone in this war zone of an economic climate
I need us to find a way to live happily ever after
            together

so let's talk
let's talk and figure out how
teach me how to be an ally to your struggle

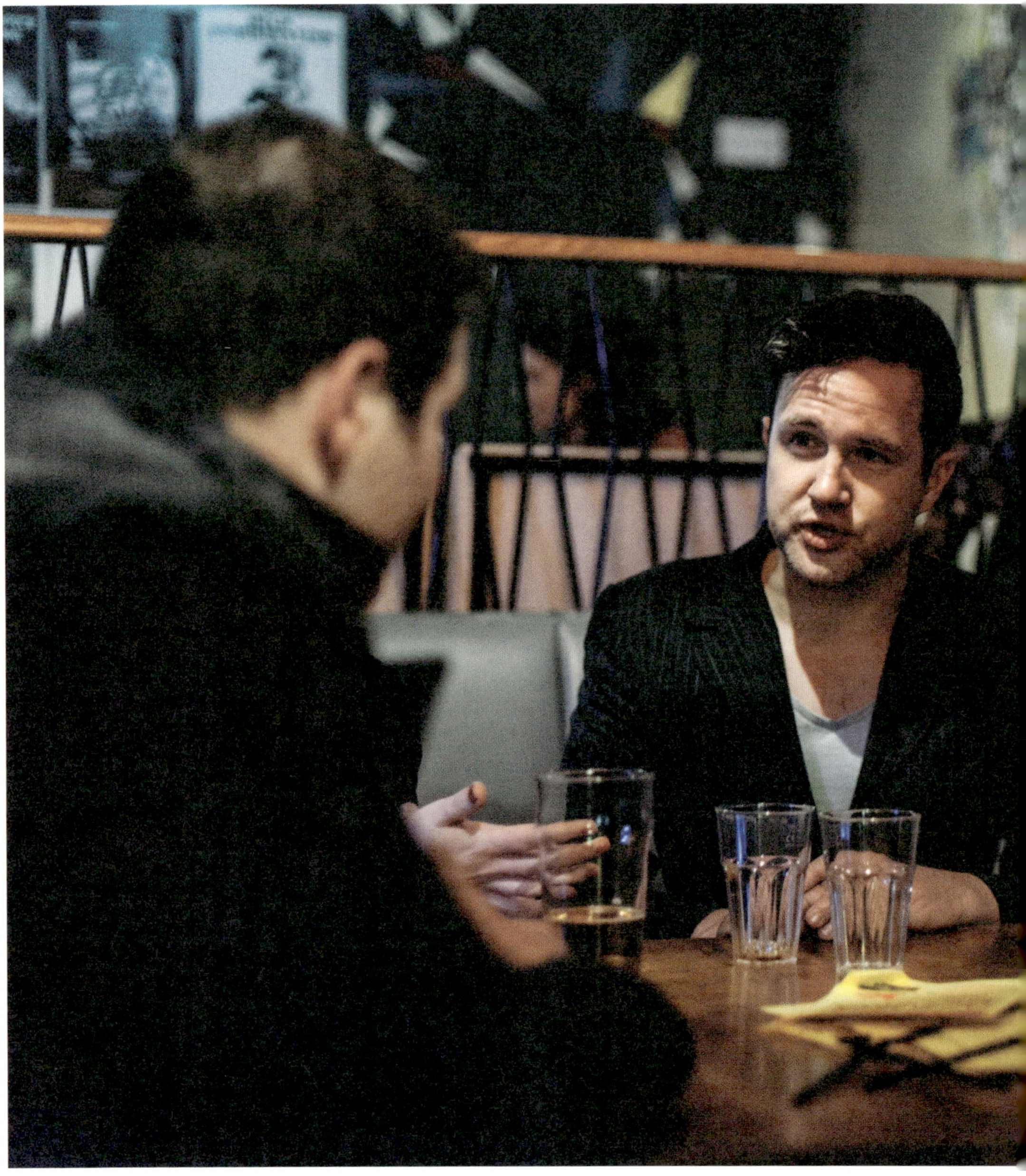

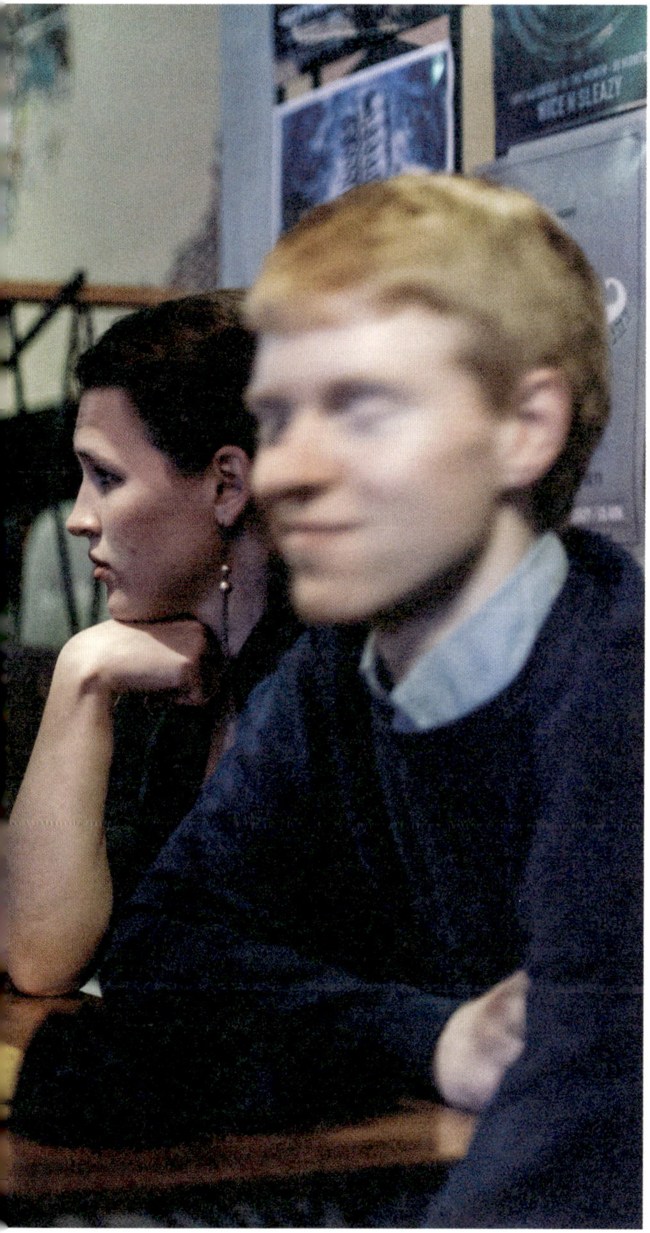

Most people aren't getting their information from Salmond, Darling, Cameron, the radio or anything else within hailing distance of a soundbite. They're getting it from each other... Every family and every workplace has become its own tiny nation-state, with all possible shades of opinion there on display.

Bella Bathurst

Extract from *Salmond and Darling squabble, but the real conversation about the Scottish referendum is elsewhere*

Taps Aff

Lacking all inhibition. A feeling of simultaneous invincibility and euphoria. See also peely wally, laldy.

With about 18 months to go to the referendum people realised this was a special, possibly unique, time, and that they could and must do what they wanted with it. Individually and collectively, inhibitions melted away and people thought and did, well, everything and anything.

What happens when the public stop listening to politicians saying 'Yes we can' and instead starts doing it themselves?

s c o t l a n d !
s c o t l a n d !
s c o t l a n d !
declare independence!
don't let them do that to you
declare independence!
don't let them do that to you!
declare independence!
don't let them do that to you!
declare independence!
don't let them do that to you!
start your own currency!
make your own stamp
protect your language

declare independence
don't let them do that to you
declare independence
don't let them do that to you

make your own flag!
raise your flag!

declare independence!
don't let them do that to you!
declare independence!
don't let them do that to you!

damn colonists
ignore their patronizing
tear off their blindfolds
open their eyes

declare independence!
don't let them do that to you!
declare independence!
don't let them do that to you!

with a flag and a trumpet
go to the top of your highest mountain!

raise your flag!

declare independence!
don't let them do that to you!
declare independence!
don't let them do that to you!

raise the flag!

Bjork

Facebook, 17 September 2014

Taps Aff

Siân Bevan

Taps Aff is the secret optimism of Scotland. It's about grabbing a glimmer of hope and laying yerself bare, ready to crinkle in rare sunlight. It's understanding that our summer isn't like everyone else's summer. It's a concept, a set of circumstances. It's an opportunity.

When given the chance last year, Scotland's soul was right there, ready to launch into a Taps Aff moment. No matter how fleeting it would turn out to be, a heartbeat of people turned to each other and picked up the hem of their inhibitions, peeling it up and back until we were there, as a group, gleaming in the warmth.

Taps Aff is confidence. It's swagger. It's a lack of fuck-giving, this is me, look if you wanna but I couldn't give a shite.

Taps Aff swings its arm around the people it loves and breathes in their ear.

Taps Aff is infectious. You might not have the baws to be the first but when you see someone with their chest oot and proud, it prickles something inside and gives you the courage to strip yerself back. One Taps Aff alone is a spectacle. When enough folk join in, it's the prudishly buttoned up who look foolish.

Taps Aff isn't perfect. It's not about sculpted bods. It's not beach body ready because it's always ready for the beach, just add sand and chips and we're there.

Taps Aff is fleeting.

When the clouds came over again, and we all put our clothes back on, there was time in the shadows. The dazed moments where we cover ourselves, arms folded awkwardly hunched as we can't believe we *did* that. People who'd never screamed slogans with passion before checked their voices for damage and went back to a normal timbre. Posters came down from windows and sad hugs stretched closely bonded friendships back to their normal distance.

Our skin was covered again but we'd all caught a bit of the sun. Maybe too much, as some of the burns felt real and sore.

And then it faded, gently. We were healthier for it. We were more confident for it. We were even able to laugh about the exuberance of it with those who'd decided to keep their jumpers on. Some of that lot called us childish, and tousled our hair saying it was for the best but you did look like you were having fun, out there with all of you dancing in the sunshine but it's cloudy now, come inside.

They didn't really understand what it was like. When it felt like we were part of something fresh and naked and scary and sweaty.

Our clothes stayed on for a while but they seem to fall off much easier now.

Taps Aff is eternal.

Once you've wriggled with warmth on your skin, there's always a part of you which wants to lay itself bare.

Taps Aff knows there will always be another sunny day.

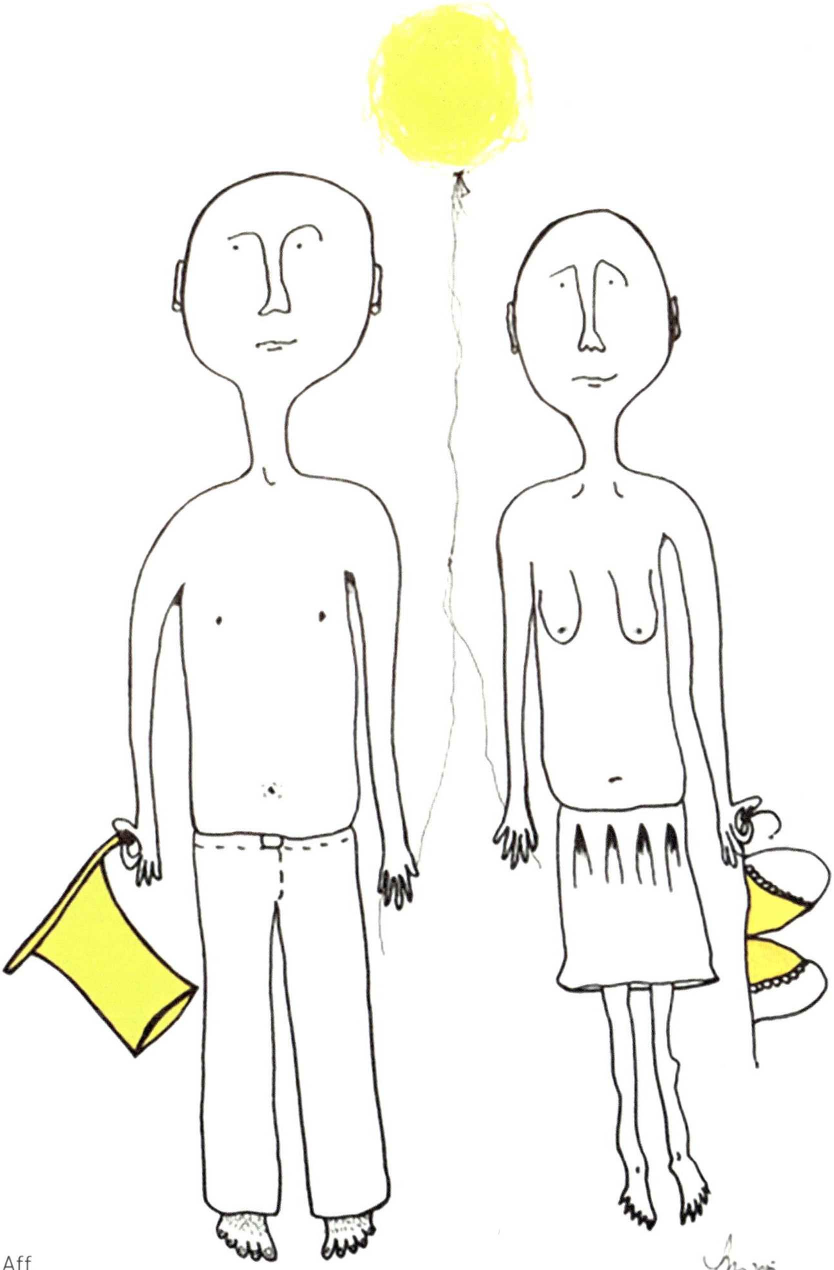

Taps Aff
Elizaveta Maltseva

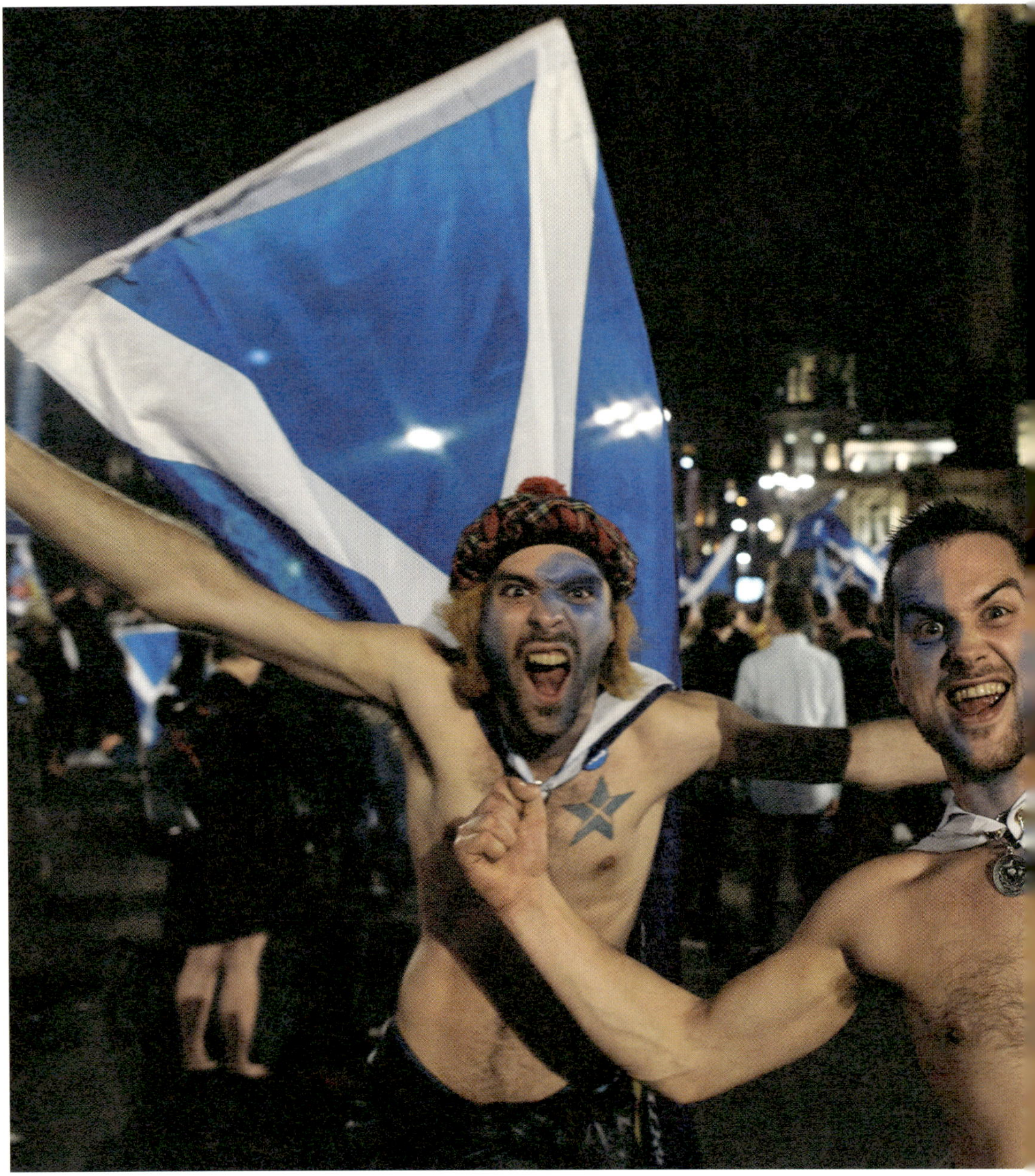

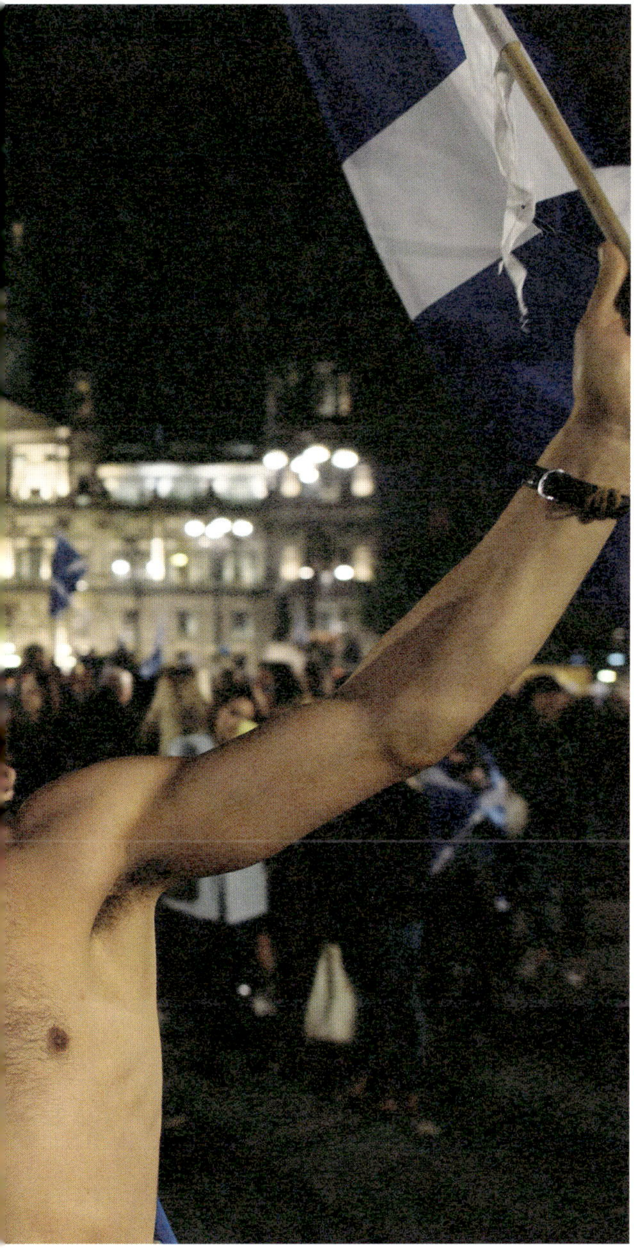

"All across Scotland people are waking up.They are rubbing their eyes, remembering this is their country and becoming angry at what it has become. If they too can have the knowledge of how we can change and the confidence that we can do it, for how much longer can the elite run our lives without our consent?"

Extract from *Common Weal: The Book*

Hoachin

Teeming with life, frenetic with activity.
"The Mile is aye hoachin in August"

The received wisdom is that we are in a post-political age where the public don't care any more. Which made the packed community centres and village halls where ordinary people across the country listened to political debate more than just a surprise.

How do we achieve real political participation and how can it change things?

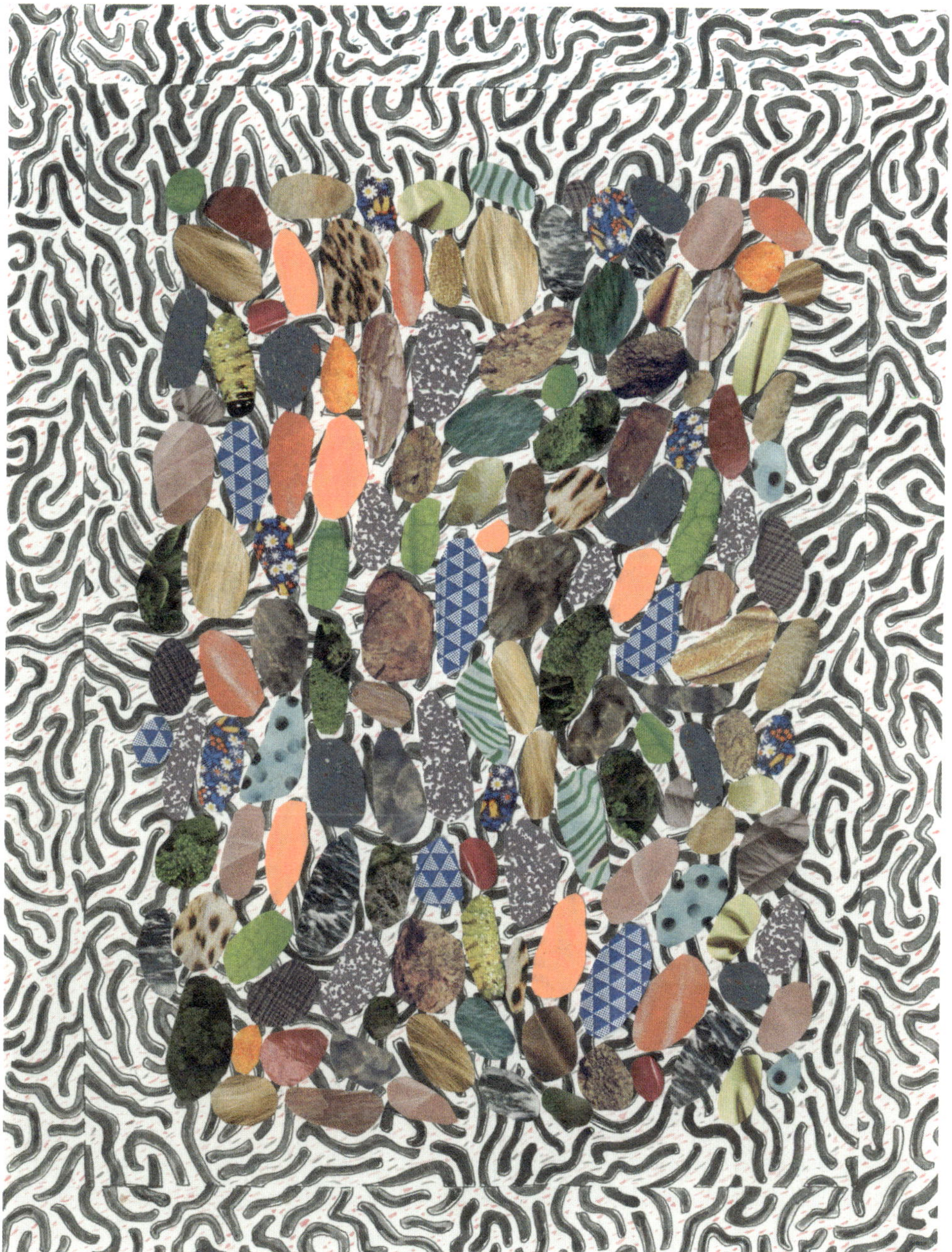

Hoachin
Suzy Lickley

Hoachin

Leela Soma

"Hoachin, aye, so it is," Maggie remarked to Rupa, as the van drove right up to the door. Rupa got the wheelchair out and helped Maggie to sit comfortably before she opened the door to the public hall. The car park was busy, the driver glad to get a disabled parking spot.

Standing room only, the town hall was overflowing. Maggie was right, it was indeed hoachin! Rupa pushed Maggie in the wheel chair, right along to the edge of the first row. They both had the SNP lanyard dangling from their necks, the dark blue against the neon yellow visibility jackets they wore. A frisson of excitable chatter was palpable as people talked to their neighbours. A few were glowering at the foes with whom they had had argued vociferously at various times during the campaign. The noise subsided as the politicians took their seats on the podium.

Vikram slid in beside Rupa and held her hand. She smiled and squeezed his hand. The evening began. The hours passed quickly with question after question as the political parties were grilled on the consequences of the Referendum. Maggie put them in a spot with her question on the rise of the food banks. The loud applause and cheers made her sit up straight and she demanded an answer.

Arguments continued as the crowd spilled out the doors at the end. Vikram and Rupa took Maggie to the van and made sure she was settled in her seat.

"Thank you, tha' was brilliant, hen." Maggie smiled sweetly at Rupa.

They waved her off and walked hand in hand towards Vikram's car.

"YOU are brilliant," Vikram planted a kiss on her cheek. Her eyes sparkled, and then she heard that distinctive cough. She moved several inches away from Vikram as if she had been stung.

Her dad stood beside the car.

It was a silent ride home. His anger, like a steel scarf tightening round her.

The wall shuddered with the impact as Rupa ran up the stairs and slammed the bedroom door. She had to escape to her haven.

'Rupa, come down at once.' Dad's voice trailed off as she stuck the Apple earbuds in. Lady Alba's 'Caught in a Bad Romance' made her giggle.

" *Naw, Naw...*

I want your weapons.

I want student fees.

I want a country run by Tory MPs.

I want your love, even if it's wrong, I like being told what I should do."

It would be mental to try something new.

Let's sit around and wait for things to improve."

She couldn't ignore the banging on the door any longer. Dad stood outside, red faced, shaking his head. He walked in and sat down heavily on the bed and looked down, dejected.

Rupa took the buds out of her ears and sat facing him.

"*Beti*, so you are running around with this old, useless guy, that *badmash*."

"I love him." Tears wet her eyelids.

"Love? You should be concentrating on your studies."

"But dad, I am studying. I've passed all my exams!"

"That ruffian, out all hours with that man! He's too old for you! No, I say no to all that canvassing nonsense with him. He's using you."

"Why do you hate him so? Anyway my support for SNP has nothing to do with him! Dad, do you know what it is like at the public meetings? Hoachin' with people. They are energised, wanting to have a stake in this country's future."

"Don't you lecture me *beti*. I've seen them all. The politicians, just like that man of yours, trying to get what they want and then abandon you."

"Dad!"

"Those politicians, the whole lot have been at the Gurdwara, the temples and the Mosques. All they want is your vote. This new party SNP is trying to get you young people to vote for them with empty promises."

"New! SNP a new party! Dad, you really don't have a clue."

"*Beti*, it is you who knows nothing. It was the United Kingdom gave me this opportunity to build my life here, when I came to Glasgow 30 years ago, to educate you and make something of my life. And you know nothing about the Partition, how our families were affected by that In India in 1947. Separation is not good."

"But Dad... listen, please, your generation still harks back to your experience of India and Pakistan. I feel not just Asian, I'm Scottish and proud of it. I love my Asian heritage but this is home for me. I feel it in my blood. Dad, you listen to the radio and TV but why don't you just come out to one of the public meetings and see what's happening around you?"

"I've been a Labour voter all my life and that will never change, and stop this gallivanting around with this old man. He's thirty! I know what is good for you. I forbid you to see him. You are too young."

"No Dad, I'm old enough to vote, old enough to get married, and do what I want! But I need your love. You brought me up after mum died...," Rupa sobbed.

He went over to her side and held her in his arms, as he had done all through her life. She rested her head on his shoulder. He ruffled her hair and planted a kiss on top of her forehead.

She moved away. Conflicting thoughts raced through her head. Vikram, Dad, the tussle that had been going on for months now. Too many thoughts 'hoachin', like Maggie had said about the public hall today. She had to make her mind up. Her freedom now, or be with her dad and allow him to run her life.

Her dad found the note when he got back from work. She had made her choice.

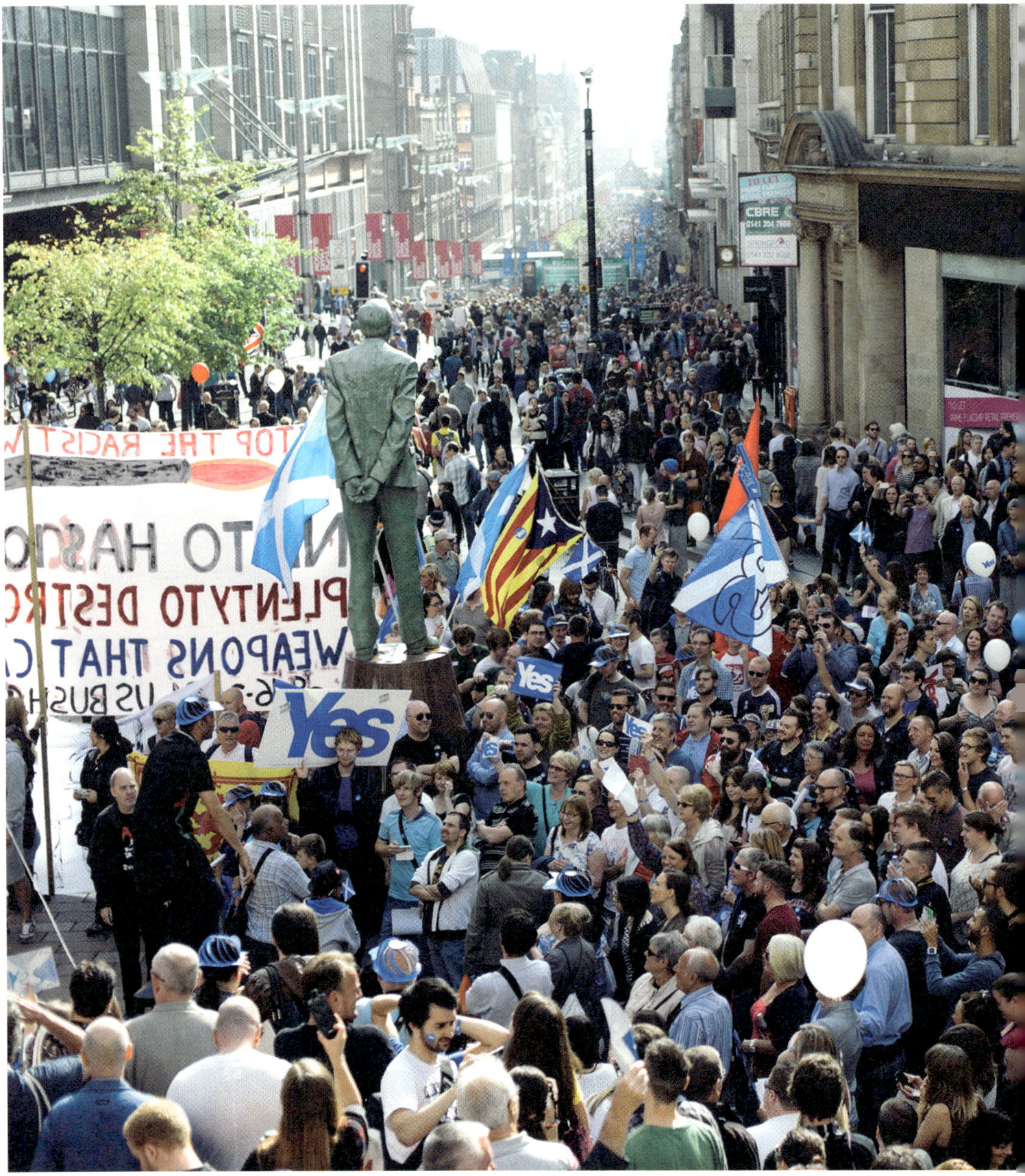
TOP THE RACIST
PLENTYTO DESTR
WEAPONS THAT
Yes
TO LET
CBRE

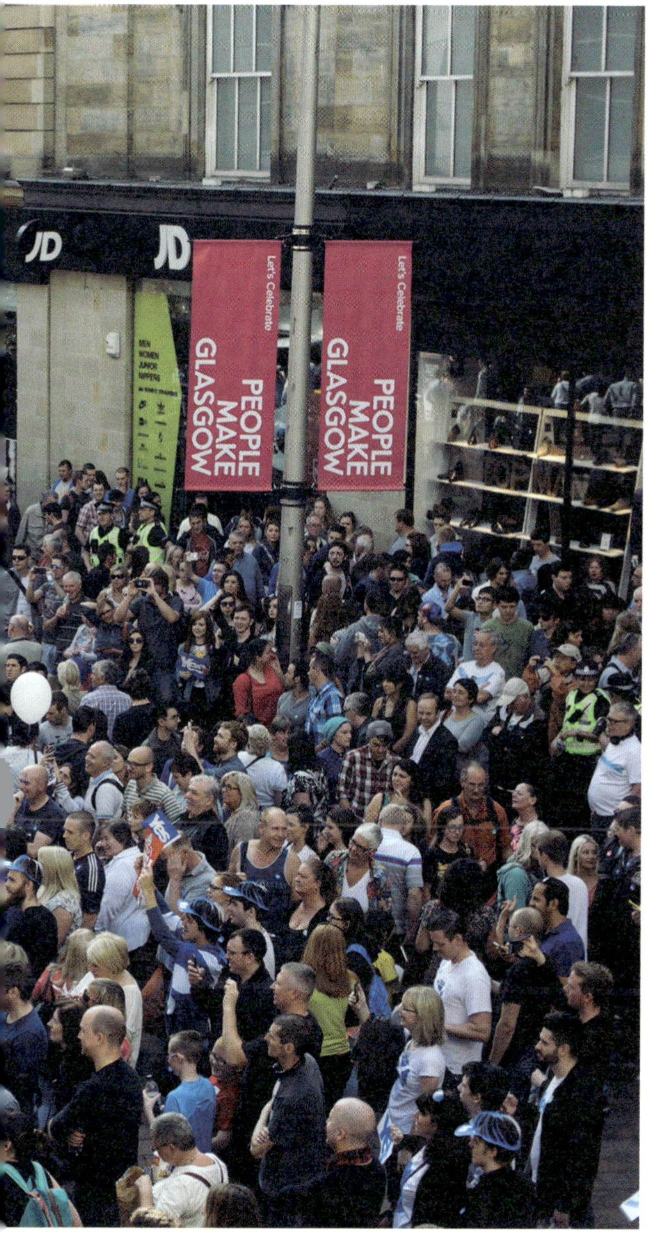

"A participatory democracy does of course have elected politicians but it also has many ways for ordinary people to participate in decision-making all the time. It designs its democracy to have the maximum opportunities for people to get involved in standing for election, whether they are in a political party or not. It brings democracy as close to the people who are affected by decisions as is possible. When decisions have to be made it involves the public in making and shaping those decisions. It is an attempt to create government by participation - where those affected by the decision are involved in the making of the decision."

Extract from *Common Weal: The Book*

Ken (v)

To know, understand, have awareness of. "Ken?"

As the referendum drew nearer, more and more people realised they weren't getting the information they wanted from the Internet—so they started to do it themselves, and get it from each other. The Scottish independence campaign has been described as one of the biggest movements of mass political self-education ever, evidenced in the pioneering new media environment in Scotland.

Is an informed, interested politically-educated population a possibility? How do we get there?

One result of the independence campaign has been that power has been exposed. Which politicians and businesses share a common interest, how the media operates and how information is distorted and ideas abused has all been opened up.

Mike Small

Extract from *An Independent Media for Scotland*

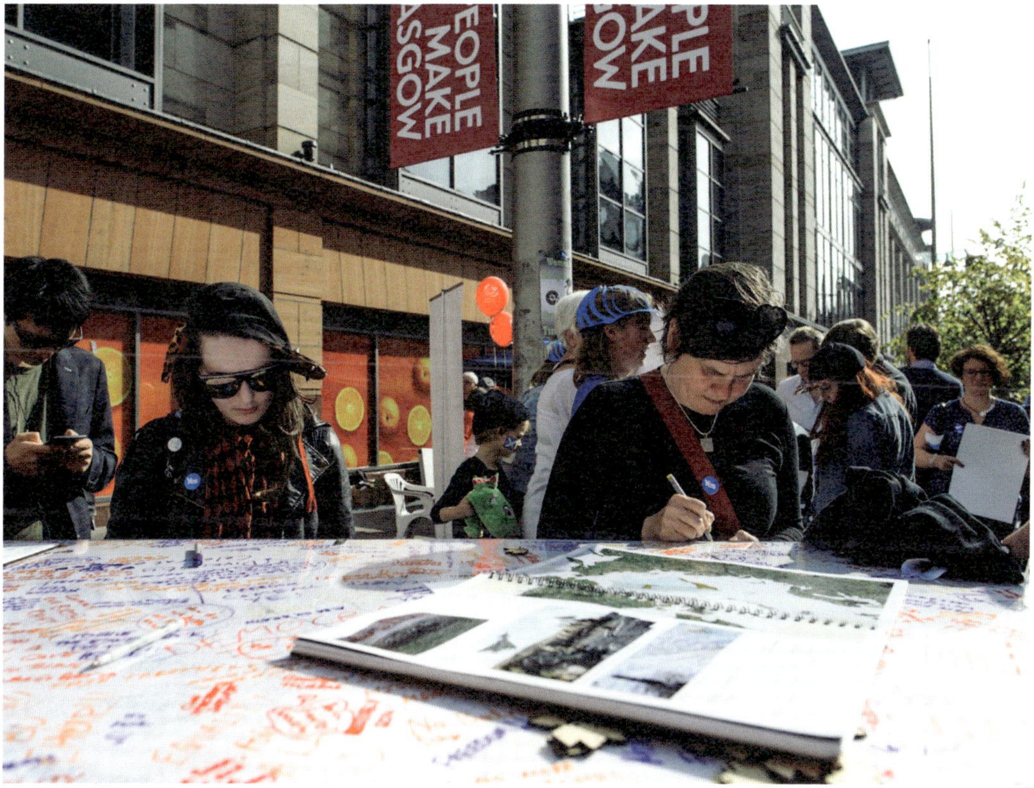

Peter McNally / Documenting Yes

Ken What? – A Confession of Love from an Egyptian Immigrant

Sara Shaarawi

Ken What?

This morning I read that part of the Italian consulate in Cairo was destroyed by a car bomb. My mother is Italian. I have been in that building countless times. I see images of the ruins of this historic building in the heart of Cairo and an influx of memories overwhelm me.

I remember waiting patiently on benches while my mother furiously mumbled and complained about Italian bureaucracy. I remember the high ceiling and the big marble staircase. At least, I think it was marble. I remember the feeling of coolness when you first enter, a relief from the heat outside.

It's strange for me to connect images I've seen of ISIS destroying faraway places to these images that are so familiar. You never imagine the big, bad wolf would ever hit this close to home. Or in this case, literally a tiny part of home.

President Sisi and his great army have announced that the situation is under control. All this does is confirm to me that nothing in Egypt is alright at the moment, and it probably won't be for a while. This attack pulls at the emotional strings I have to the city of Cairo, and evokes an instant urge to go back. But unlike the other times 'shit went down' in Egypt, this time I don't actually contemplate going back.

Ken What?

I didn't choose Scotland the first time around. It just happened. Or for those of you more inclined to mystical explanations: Scotland chose me. When I applied for postgraduate studies, out of the institutions which accepted me, Edinburgh University was simply the most economical option. When asked why I chose Scotland at the time, I just shrugged and said I wanted to be somewhere in Europe. As an afterthought I added that I liked the accents. It would take me at least a year to realise that the Scottish accent wasn't just an accent. That's after I slowly realised that Scotland was not England, and that the UK was not Europe, and that Europe, in fact, was not Europe.

In Egypt, we call all countries that are not Egypt 'the countries on the outside'. The saying always evoked a sense of freedom in travelling abroad. And for Egyptians it is very true, because the quest for a visa is not an easy one. I, however, was lucky to be born to an Italian mother, another event which I did not choose, but one which granted me a freedom that is the envy of those belonging to the country I grew up in. A freedom which, I have to say, is taken for granted in most EU countries.

Ken What?

I did choose Scotland the second time around. After a dizzying year of moving every four months to a different European country, I finally graduated with a second masters degree. I had to choose where I would become an adult. And so I chose Scotland.

People always ask me what Scotland is like and my first response is always: 'The weather is shit and the food is horrible.' I enjoy seeing the confused looks on people's faces, these two features being essential to day-to-day life. Then I tell them, 'But it makes up for it.' Yes, the weather is muggy, but the people are vibrant and there's always a story to be heard or a song to be sung or a deep, drunken conversation to be had. And yes, the food is horrible at first, but you get used to it. Then you crave it. I never thought I would ever enjoy eating a scotch pie; now I have one almost every week. Most of all, there is community here and I never felt so welcomed anywhere else in my life.

I was excited to be moving back in the year the referendum on independence was going to take place. And when I found out that I also had a vote, that's when I knew that this country was doing something right. At the time I got into several discussions about my eligibility to vote. Only people outside of Scotland believed I didn't have that right because I wasn't Scottish. To this day I still challenge that statement and here's why:

I now refer to England as 'down south.'

I now wear a t-shirt in fifteen degree weather.

I now know what Buckfast is and what it can do.

I can now understand the lyrics to Hector Bizerk's rap songs.

And, I repeat, I now eat a scotch pie almost every week.

I voted in the referendum, because this is where I choose to call home. And, rightfully so, my home gave me a right to vote. So to all those people who questioned my legitimacy to vote due to my lack of Scottishness, I will take this opportunity to say: get tae fuck!

Ken What?

Scotland is where I became a writer. It is where I learned to tell stories, where I began to frame my experiences, where I realised that people might actually be interested in what I have to say. Scotland is where I realised that failure is not the end of the world. It's where I learned that a casual act of kindness towards a stranger can change a person's life. Scotland is the place where I finally accepted that I'm a mongrel, and it's something to celebrate not resent.

Ken What?

Ken is the first Scots word I ever learned. I learned it when I first moved back to Scotland, it was the moment I realised it's not that Scottish people have a difficult accent, it's that they use entirely different words. Theoretically, I knew that Scots existed, and academics in Edinburgh University had tried to explain to me the complexity of language in Scotland, obviously to no avail. It took me a long time to finally HEAR the words. And funnily enough, it began with 'ken', which I must confess I misheard at first.

Instead of 'ken' I heard 'care', much to the frustration of the person speaking to me. But I like how I misheard it. So now, forever engraved in the Scottish makeup my language is acquiring, *ken* means 'know' with just a touch of 'care'; exactly how I feel about this place, a yearning to know more that stems from deep, mutual care. And that's why, as much as I love Cairo, I don't contemplate leaving anymore. Ken what I mean?

Ken
Mark Campbell

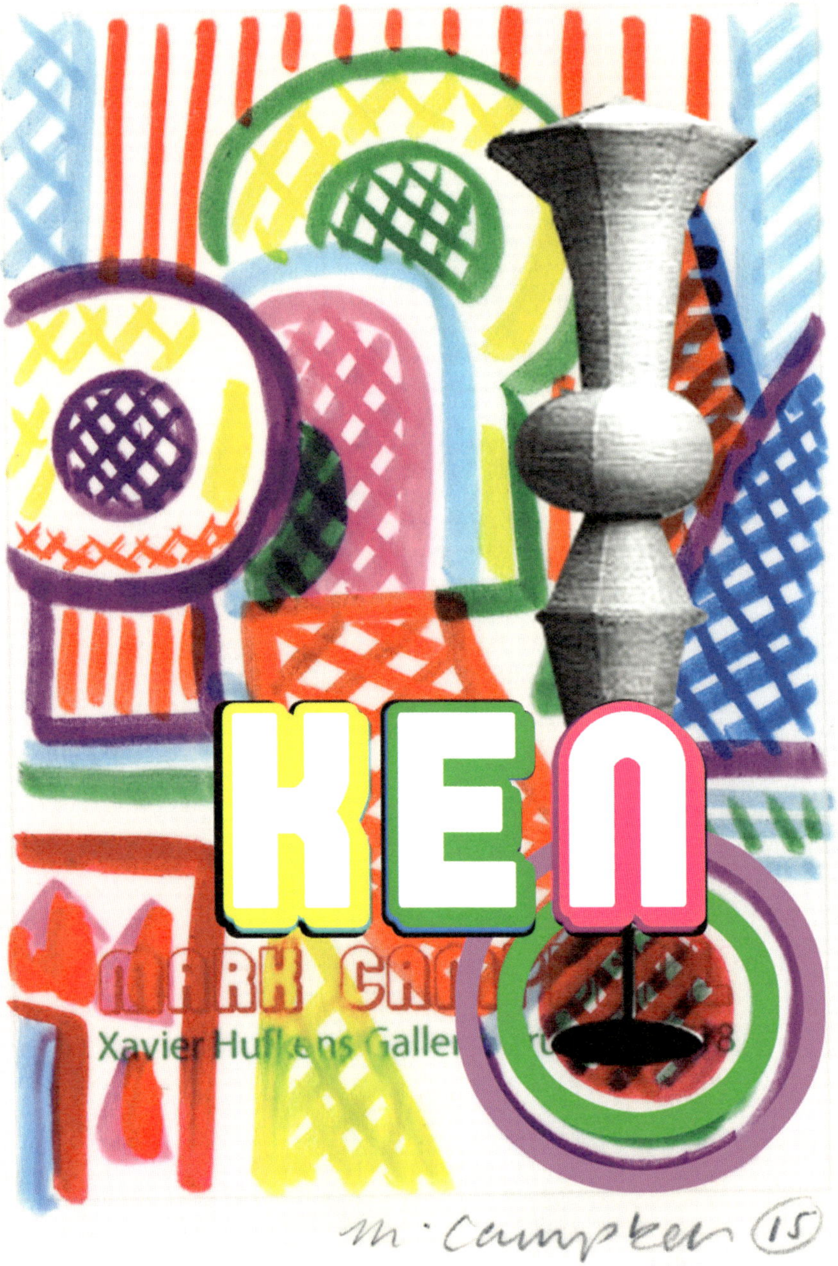

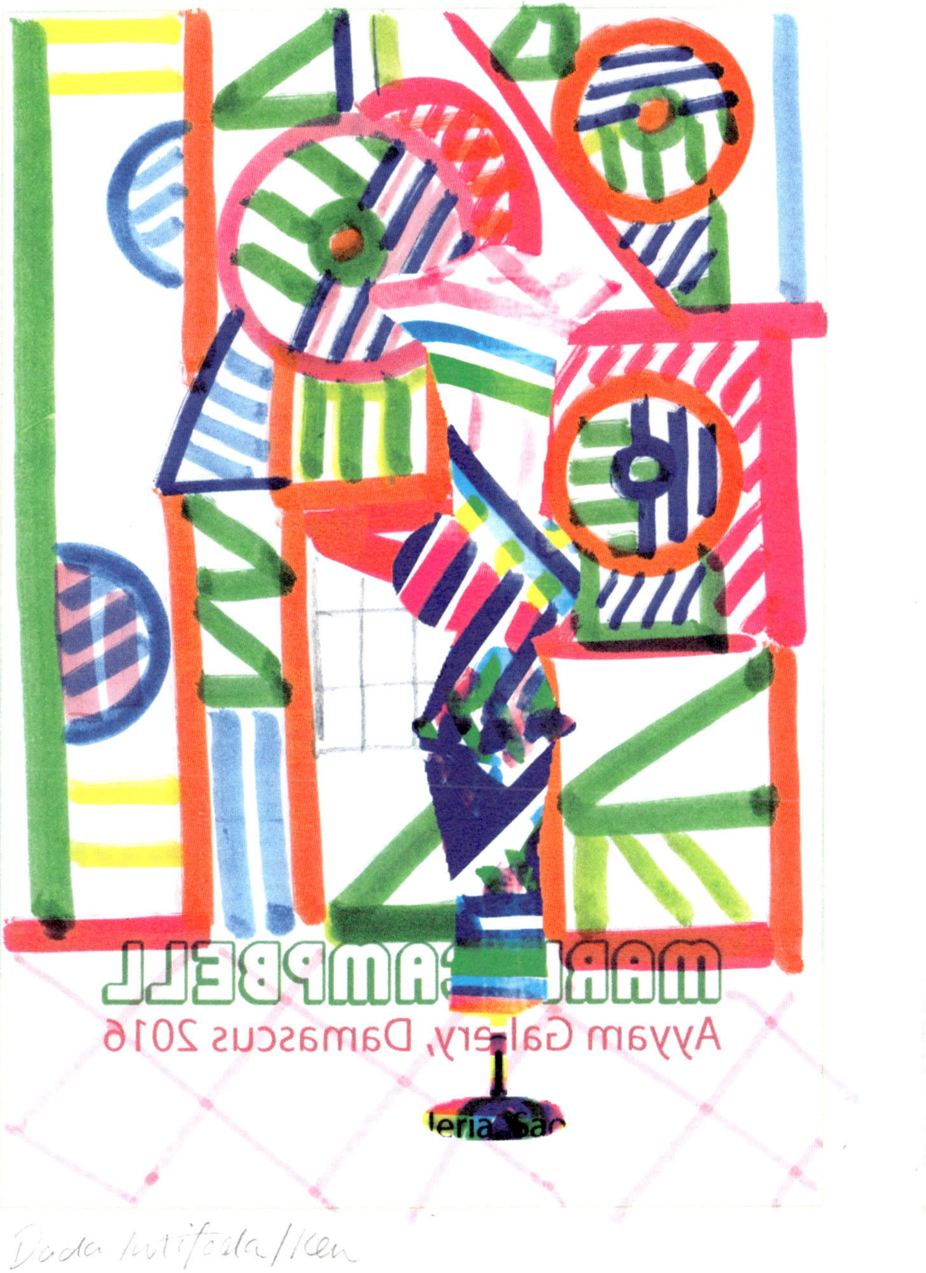
Dada Intifada/Ken

Rammy

An altercation, fracas, brawl. Often with the inclusion of a number of participants. See also; stooshie, stramash, square go.

The independence campaign was diverse and spoke with many voices from across the political spectrum. What began as a stale prospectus became a chaotic battle of ideas, art and activism from every nook of our society.

We've become so used to monolithic politics that lots of people having their own ideas at first seemed shocking. How do we change that?

Rammy
Samantha McPherson

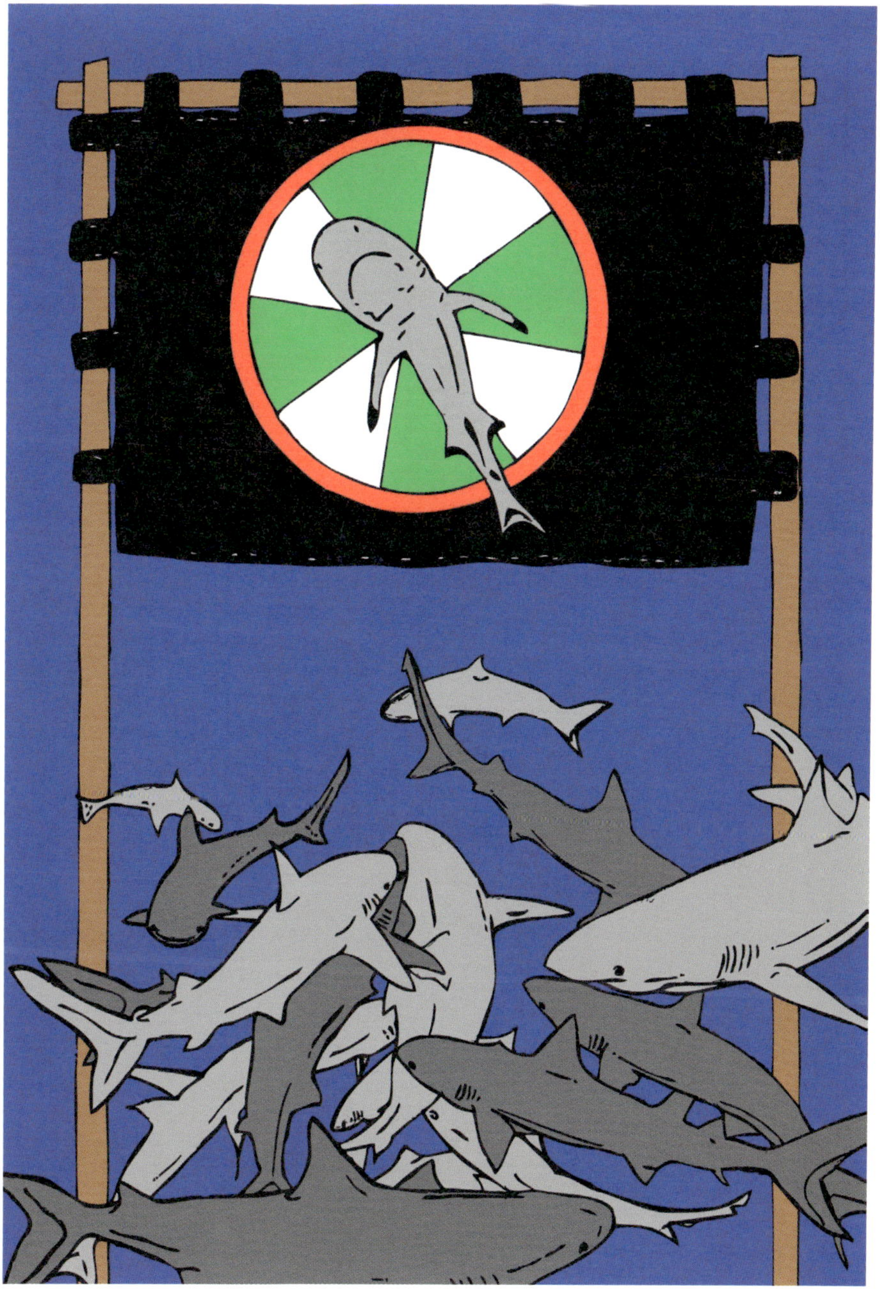

Rammy
Peter Arnott

A rammy is something you overhear, to my mind. It's an argument longer on heat than light. Less a dialectic...more a lot of shouting. The kind of thing that happens when you put a Labour MSP and and SNP MSP in the same room together...if there's anybody watching. Two voices that sound almost identical yelling over each other about which one gets to occupy the exact same Scots half acre of space on the centre left, over which one of them is "real", over which one of them is "progressive" and most noisily sterile of all...over which one of the two tiresome tumshies is more "Scottish". Not only can't they hear what the other one is saying, we can't hear them either, which may often be a blessing. God save us.

But what, I wonder, is the difference between a rammy and a stooshie...let alone a stramash? When does guid Scots flyting shade into...say... Cybernat abuse? Is it simply that we have a lot of words for "argument" in the same way that the Inuits have a lot of words for snow?

(Not that we're not weather conscious linguistically. I've a fell driech smoor oot ben ma windae the noo)

And is it really true that Scottish Cyberspace is a more abusive arena than any other corner of the internet? Has social (and anti-social) media been good for us? (Is it good for me to have John McTernan's Twitter tag handy when I feel like having a self-righteous, snide wee dig at the nihilistic Blairite whose instumentalist myopia so neatly synthesises the defeatist lack of values that ... and that's me over the 140 characters.)

It's partly because the question we were asked last year was between a Yes and a No.
I think the campaign got a lot of energy ... and a lack of thought ... from being focussed on a binary question in an analog world. Any black and white and on and off question like that gets both strength and weakness from being sufficiently stupid as to be able to mean almost anything to almost anybody. While it meant that what are called "broad churches" could argue together their two sides of the case it also cemented two "left-ish" cultures into utter mutual incomprehension which played into what was already not the most conducive of argumentative paradigms for mutual persuasion and enlightenment.

And the New Normal ... with our 56 personally impressive but arithmetically irrelevant MPs... with Labour seemingly determined to learn nothing and the SNP not feeling they really have to learn anything either, thanks ... and George Osborne's budget from a Dickens novel now defining the economic ground in which any oppositional voices are going to have to operate ... seems less than ever an arena for the imagination. There is a disturbing familiarity to the way that the SNP are becoming unexamined civic leaders in exactly the same way that the Labour Party used to be. (As were, before that, the Unionists, and before that the Dundas brothers if you want to delve that deeply into the Caledonian historical psyche.)

This is where one of the accidental by-products of that moment of sudden, focussed possibility last year comes in. The one thing about the Scottish zeitgeist that has changed irrevocably, it seems to me, no matter which side of the binary argument you were on, is that, no matter what the constitution says, there has been a transfer of psychological sovereignty. We may have chosen NOT to become independent, but WE chose, and the choice remains ours. We come from a culture that has been voluntarily subordinate since at least the 18th Century. Not any more.

And the first target of our new self confidence might just be that we demand better of our Lairds and Maisters than another continued rammy; that we use the new found sovereignty we feel, I think, in constitutional matters, and apply that confidence, that sense of self rule in economics, housing, education, health, fiscal policy .. even .. God help us .. the arts.

And start to put an argument where the rammy was.

To Mairi

thanks for coming!

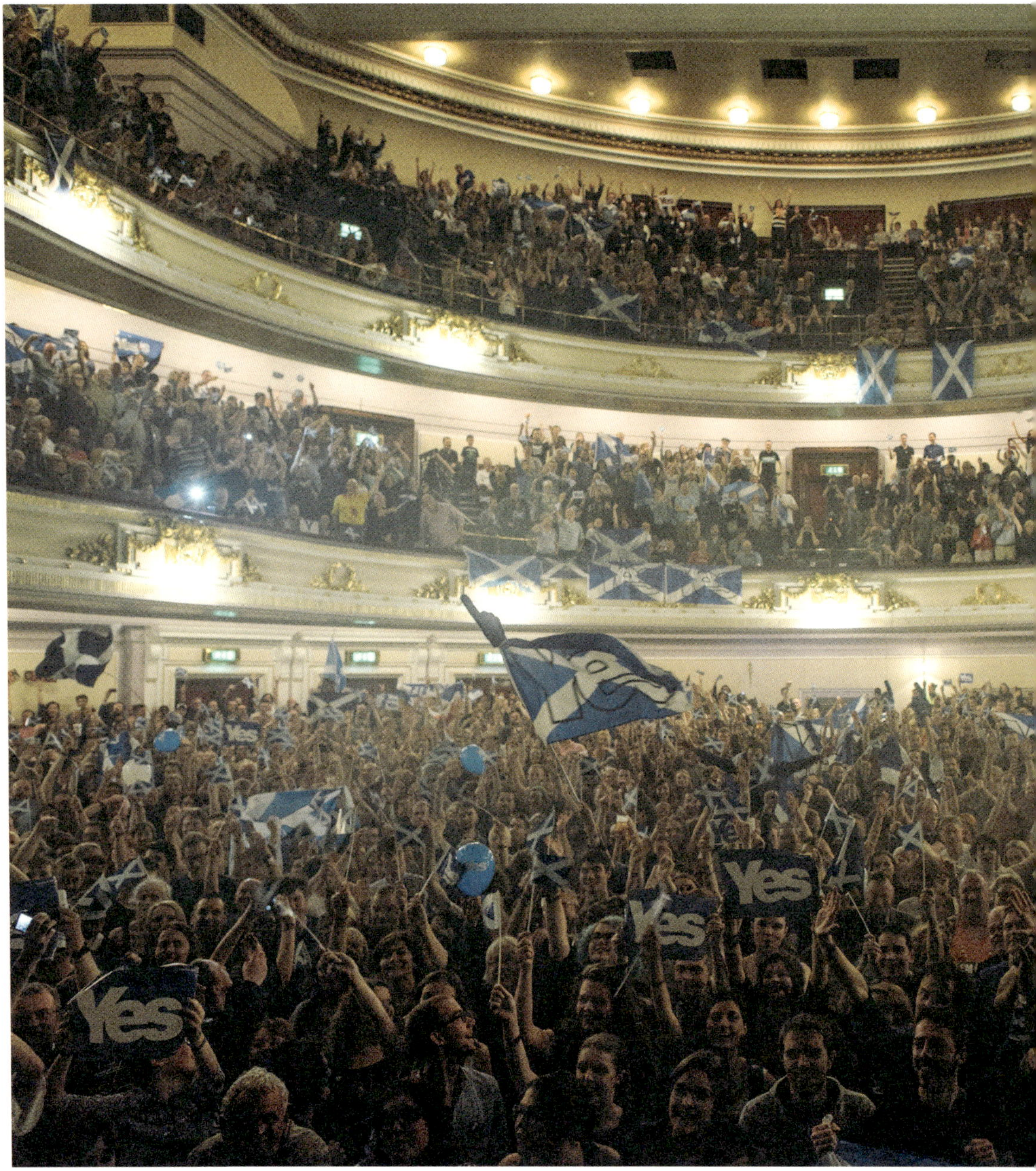
Yes
Yes
Yes
Yes

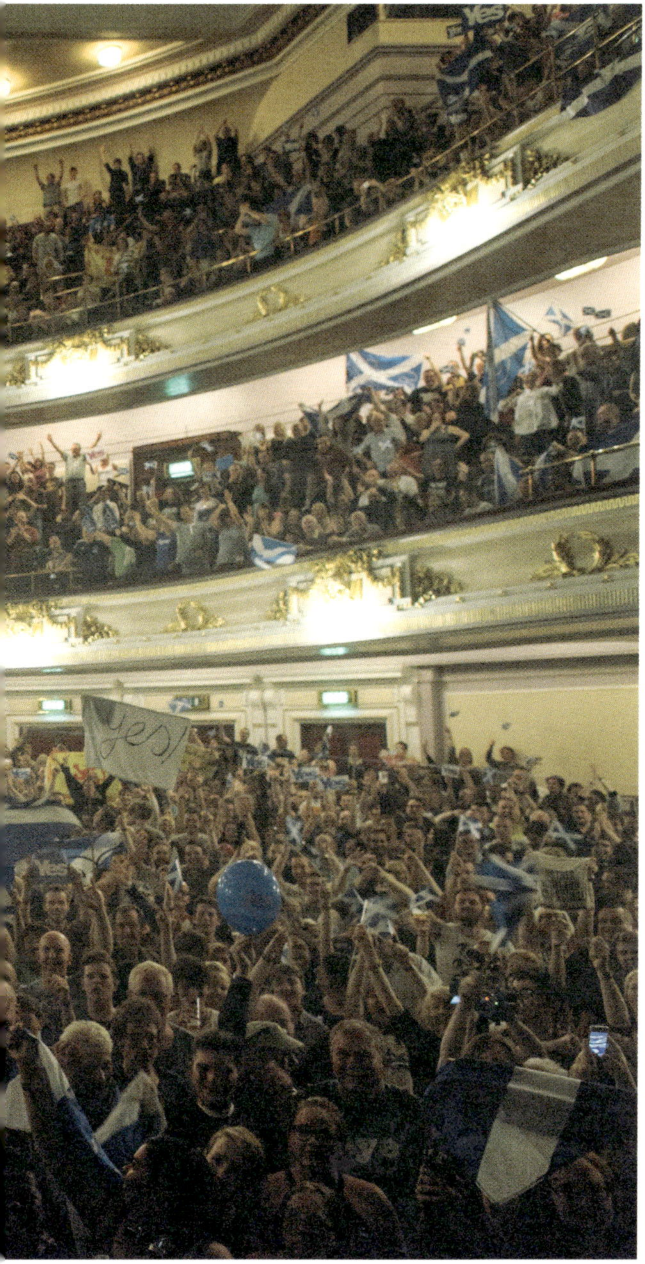

With independence We start a new era, when Scots in their own country are beholden to no one, and need ask permission of no one for policies the people need.

No more inferiority, no more minority status, no more accusations about holding out a begging bowl. A new start, when we think new thoughts, embrace new ideas and use the power that lies within us, to change things for the better, and forever.

In place of fear we can create a nation that is proud, self-confident, prosperous, where working people will have the opportunity to quickly build a fair, and just society.

Jim Sillars

Extract from *In Place of Fear*

Bide (v)

To stay, linger, inhabit, or remain. Alternatively, to infer trust or reliance on an intimate. "Bide a wee with me".

In the end, the independence campaign was about both the place we live and the society we want to be a part of. Where we stay, how we live, who we are; these topics were dissected again and again throughout the campaign.

Was the independence campaign nationalist? What was the role of identity and place?

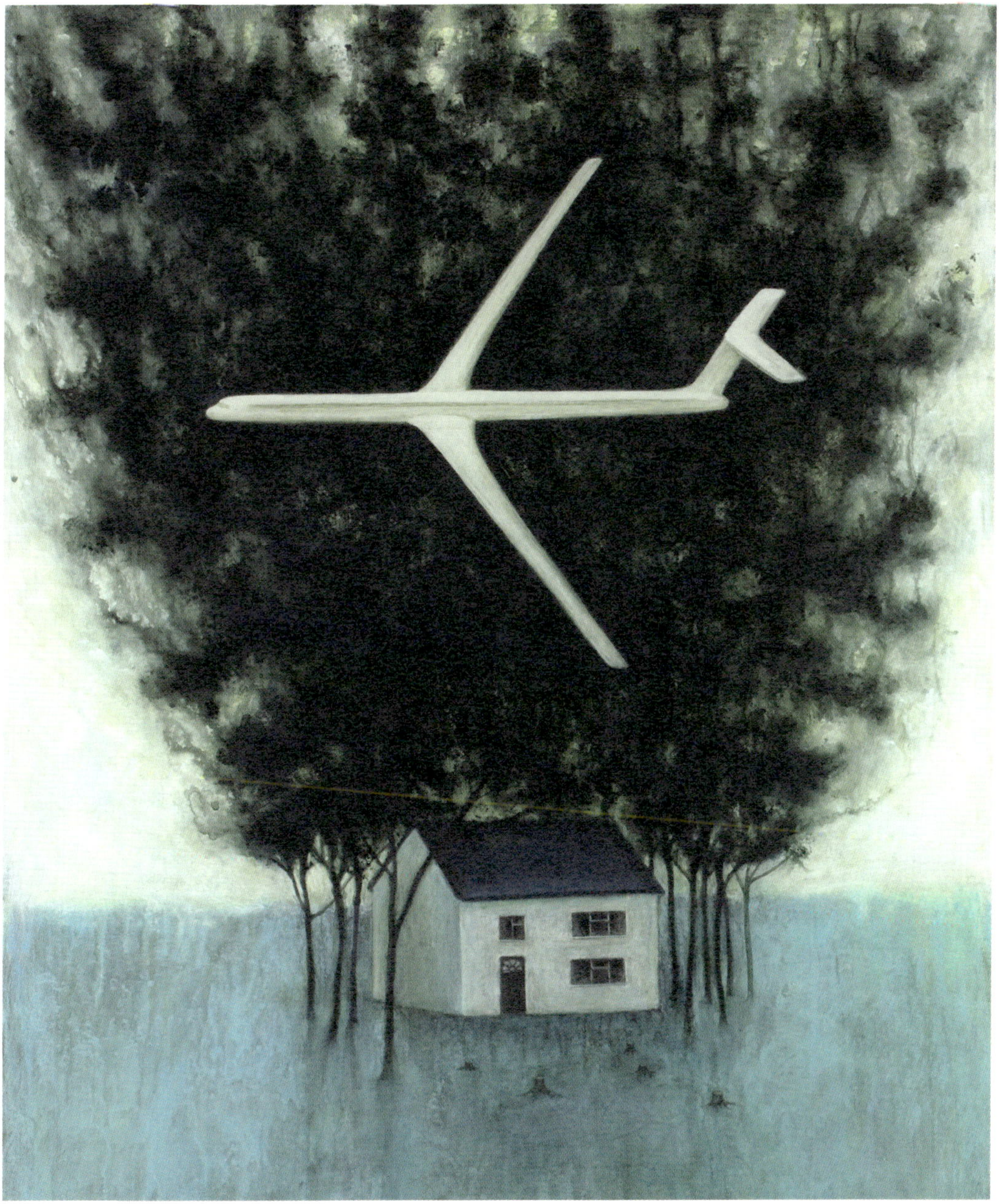

Bide
Alasdair Wallace

Bide: a triptych

Katie Gallogly-Swan

On origins.

We all have a founding myth of who we are. It normally begins with the story of our parents, or the stories of their parents, and the understanding that the ripples of serendipity that allowed their collision, also determined – to differing extents – the way we conceive of and participate in the world.

This myth is simultaneously a justification for behaviour and a verification of purpose and meaning; a means of making sense of the meanderings and marathons of our lives.

But these personal myths cannot escape the primordial soup of context. The collection of stories that bind societies together, or seismically divide them, all eddy into collectively recognised understandings of communities, cities, countries, and continents.

We are connected through these overlapping and sometimes contradictory belief systems as agents within them, navigating our own identities and participating in their perpetuation.

They stretch out to the ends of the earth, ripples expanding, contracting, and mutating into new waves. While our interpretations of these stories change with time, the only thing that remains constant is the existence of the boundaries between the "us" and the "them".

These inevitably connected founding myths are not always rational, but they are anything but trivial. They are the very fragments of our perception of self and world.

Conversations in Glasgow

1. First date

So where are you from?
The north, Inverness way.
Scotland? That's no a Scottish accent ah hear.
Well my parents weren't born in Scotland.
But you were?
No I wasn't born here but have grown up here since I was about 4.
Oh so you're not Scottish.

2. Two colleagues bond

Been here long?
Glasgow, born and bred.
Aye, I've been working here for about 14 years, it's a great city. Can't imagine living anywhere else.
Aw aye? I moved away for work near twenty year ago, but I moved back last year.
I bet a lot's changed since you left, eh?
Aw totally different city, man! Pure changed.
And are you settling in okay?
Well, aye. Tons of stuff going on. Great to be near ma family an' all that.
Why did you move back?
Referendum: I wanted my vote to count.
That's dedication. I don't need to guess what you voted!
Och aye, it was an obvious decision.
[Uneasy laughter] Suppose that depends–
–Aye if yer a Tory! Where are you from again?

3. In the playground

You're not that Scottish. You don't even like Irn Bru.

4. Family dinner

Scotland is just a more left wing place. We've always had a strong socialist legacy. You know, Jimmy Reid and the shipyards and that.
Well, what about Blair?
What about Blair?

Bowie or Bragg?
Harry or Renton?
Noam or Niall?

White man or white man?
Binary or binary?

Profile of a Scot

Sex	Female
Date of Birth	16/02/1991
Birthplace	Bellshill Maternity Hospital
Blood Type	O+
Noticeable Features	Birth mark on left rib cage
Allergies	N/A
Height	5′5″
Weight	60kg
Hair Colour	Ash
Eye Colour	Green/Grey
Shoe Size	UK 4
Dress Size	UK 10
Religion	N/A
Marital Status	Co-habitant
Number of Dependents	0
Interests	Anthropology, linguistics, feminism, sustainable living/eating, sharks
Hobbies	Running, cycling, knitting, tea, cooking
Favourite Colour	Green
Favourite Food	Pistachios, icing
Biggest Fear	Infertility
Biggest Triumph	Falling in love

Bide a wee with me, in ma
wee
twee
hame.

But as post (military) imperial, welfare state Britain declined, what I've also learned, and, like many Scots, am constantly having reinforced, is that a lot of what I believed to be 'Britishness' was really just another term for 'Englishness'...This English appropriation of Britishness, what Stuart Hall calls 'an assumed Englishness, which always negotiates against difference', is now a powerful hegemonic force, which serves this state. In the past, when that 'Britishness' was formed by imperial and industrial expansion, and the esprit de corps engendered by WW1 and WW2 and the creation of a welfare state, it was largely an inclusive concept. Then, this 'assumed Englishness' was only a minor irritant to Scots. In the context of these islands now being a 'sales territory' in a globalized, monolithic, neo-liberal economic order, it becomes a far more sinister, inherently marginalizing force.

Irvine Welsh

Extract from *Scottish Independence and British Unity*

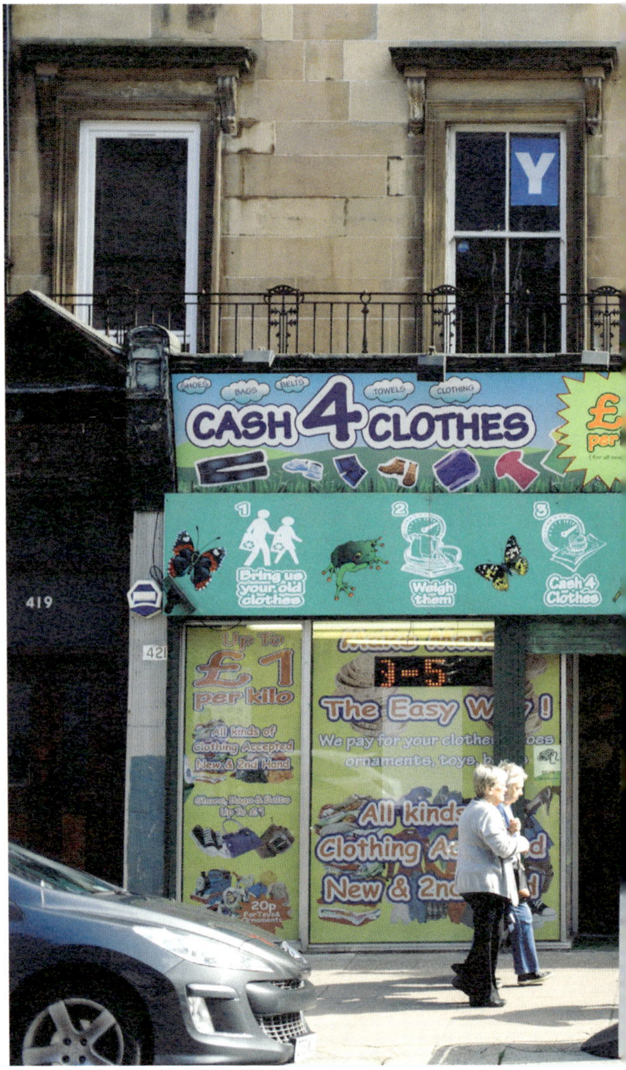
Y
CASH 4 CLOTHES
Bring us your old clothes
Weigh them
Cash 4 Clothes
419
£1 per kilo
All kinds of Clothing Accepted New & 2nd Hand

Peter McNally / Documenting Yes

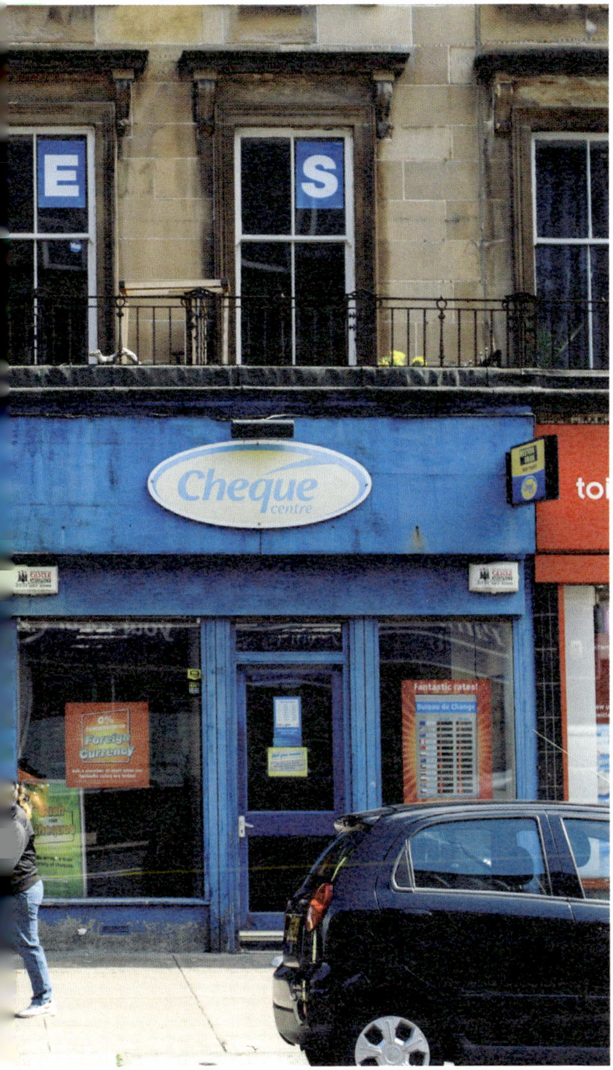

In 1999, something remarkable took place. The ownership of 26 iconic properties such as Edinburgh Castle, Stirling Castle, Linlithgow Palace, Holyrood Park, Arbroath Abbey and Dunfermline Palace were transferred by the Crown Estate Commissioners to the Secretary of State for Scotland (within a few months Scottish Ministers then took over ownership). Quite why this was done is not entirely clear but the symbolism was evident (despite there never having been any publicity about this extraordinary dowry to devolution). The Crown Estate Commissioners appeared to believe that such properties were more appropriately held by representatives of the Scottish people.

Andy Wightman

Extract from *Balmoral Buyout*

Scunnered

A profound combination of irked, disappointed and weary, such that the subject requires change from the source of such feelings.

If you spoke to many of the most active members of the campaign they would tell you that it was not nation or identity that drove their impassioned stance, but anger at the society Westminster had created with no change in sight.

Was the independence campaign anti-nationalist? Was it really driven by anger at a political system rather than identity?

There is only one thing at which any place excels – being itself. And there is only one set of people who fully understand that- the people who live there. Right now capable people all across Scotland can only stand and survey the failing public facades of their local lives.

At a meeting set up to counter decline in historic Linlithgow, I was again urging self-help. A business man told me local efforts had got nowhere – symbolized by a non-functioning light bulb in an nearby bypass.

"The council say they'll fix it, but every time I walk home, the light's not working. Maybe it's kids. Maybe they don't even change the bulb. When I complain they say it costs too much to send a workman out. So what happens? Nothing? Why do I pay council tax if the council can't even keep an underpass lit?"

"So why don't you change the light bulb yourself?"

"What?"

"Change it yourself if it annoys you so much."

"It's not my job – why should I?"

"Listen to yourself. You are consumed with anger over a £1 light bulb."

"Change it, act, do something, take charge."

There was laughter, a release of tension and then a resigned shake of the head.

"I can't. They'll prosecute me for interfering with council property." Mr Lightbulb was probably right. This is the simmering rage and wasted energy that lies at the heart of almost every local community. Little things cannot be fixed by capable local people. New ideas cannot be tried out. The people elected and employed to make decisions about the most important and intimate aspects of life are generally strangers.

Lesley Riddoch

Extract from *Blossom*

Scotland Waiting

Bashabi Fraser

This cargo of people with dreams
is stilled into inaction
trapped for now like a painted ship
upon a painted ocean

The wind has dropped
The moon is listless
The waves lie supine
in distress.

The moon, the sea and earth
are scunnered
as winds and tides of change subside
But from the depths
of an urgent core
a drumbeat pulses a fresh tide

Scunnered
Dominic Snyder

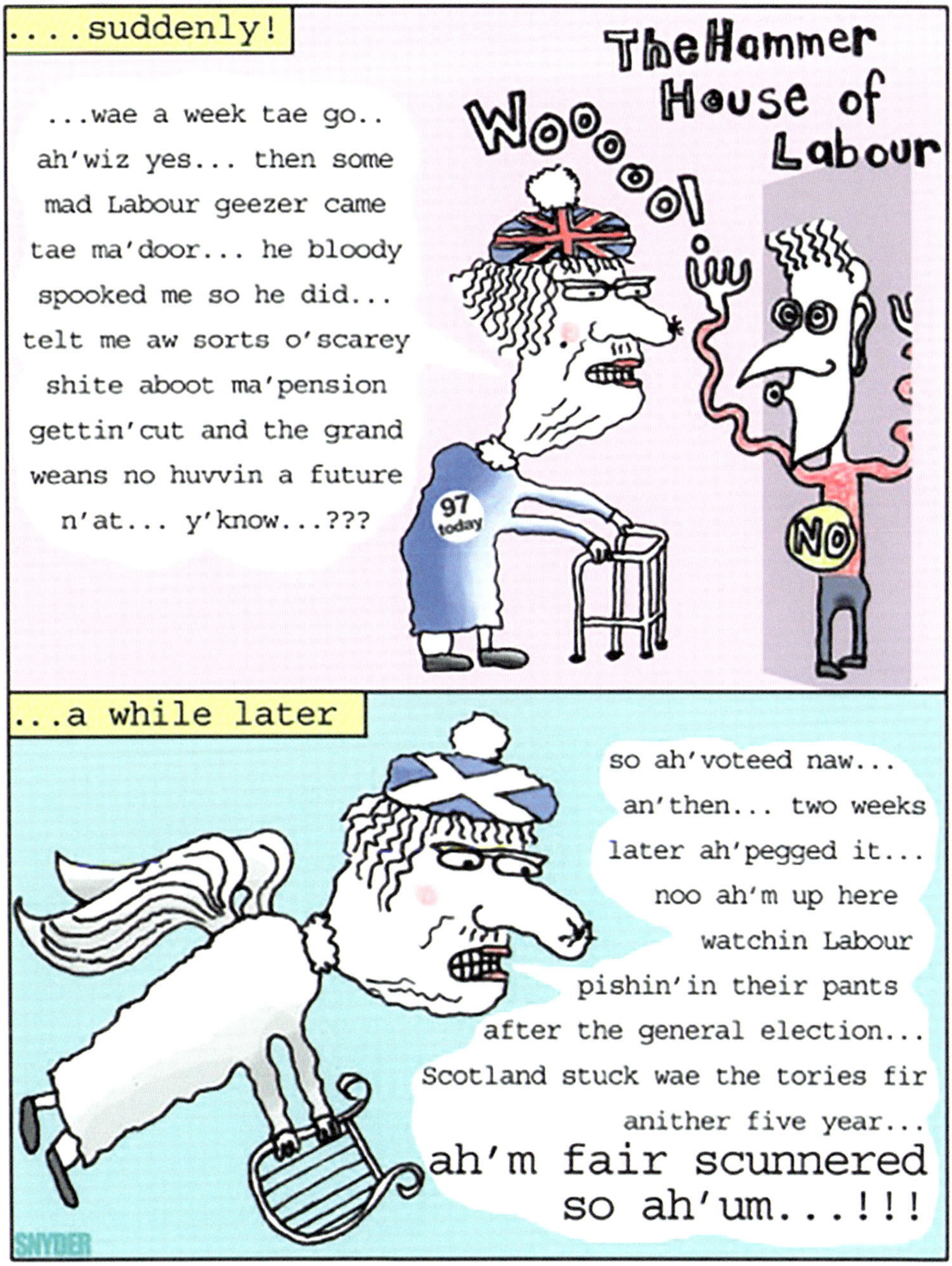
....suddenly!
...wae a week tae go.. ah'wiz yes... then some mad Labour geezer came tae ma'door... he bloody spooked me so he did... telt me aw sorts o'scarey shite aboot ma'pension gettin'cut and the grand weans no huvvin a future n'at... y'know...???
TheHammer House of Labour
Wooooool
97 today
NO
...a while later
so ah'voteed naw... an'then... two weeks later ah'pegged it... noo ah'm up here watchin Labour pishin'in their pants after the general election... Scotland stuck wae the tories fir anither five year...
ah'm fair scunnered so ah'um...!!!
SNYDER

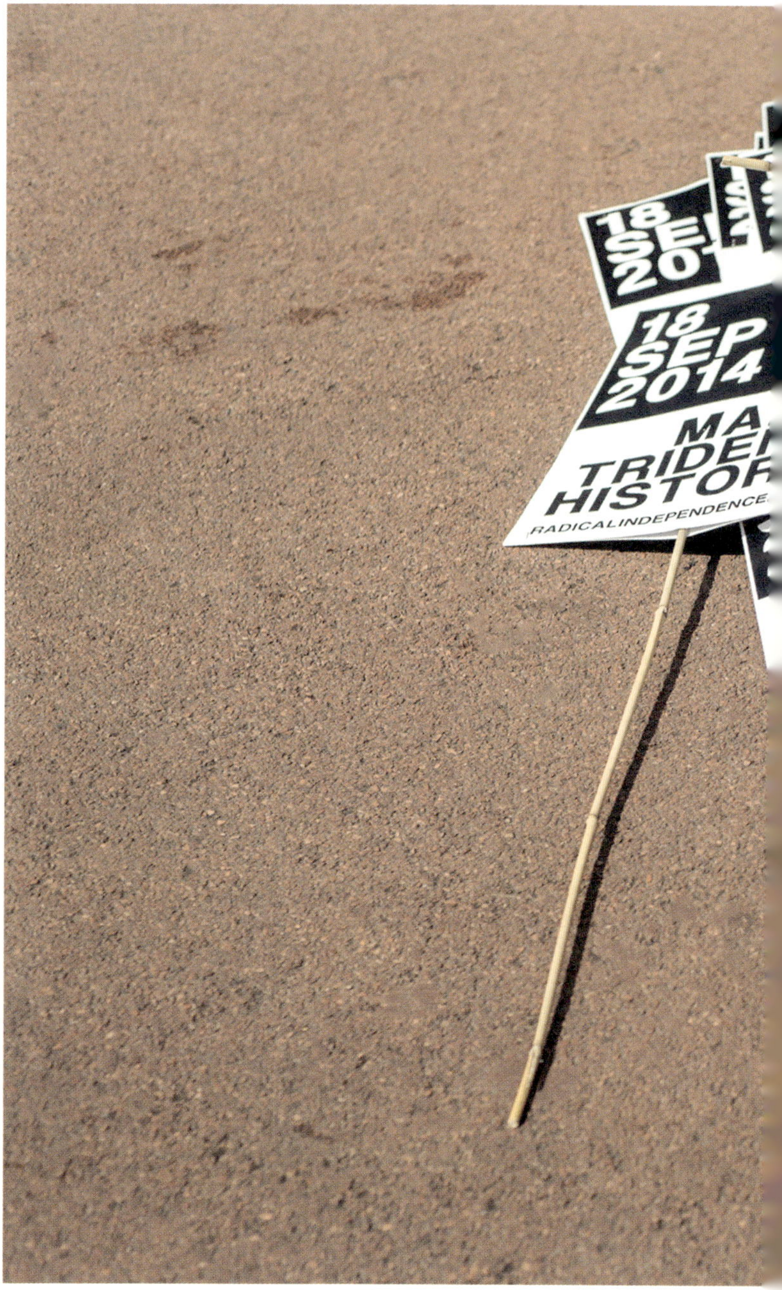
18
SEP
2014

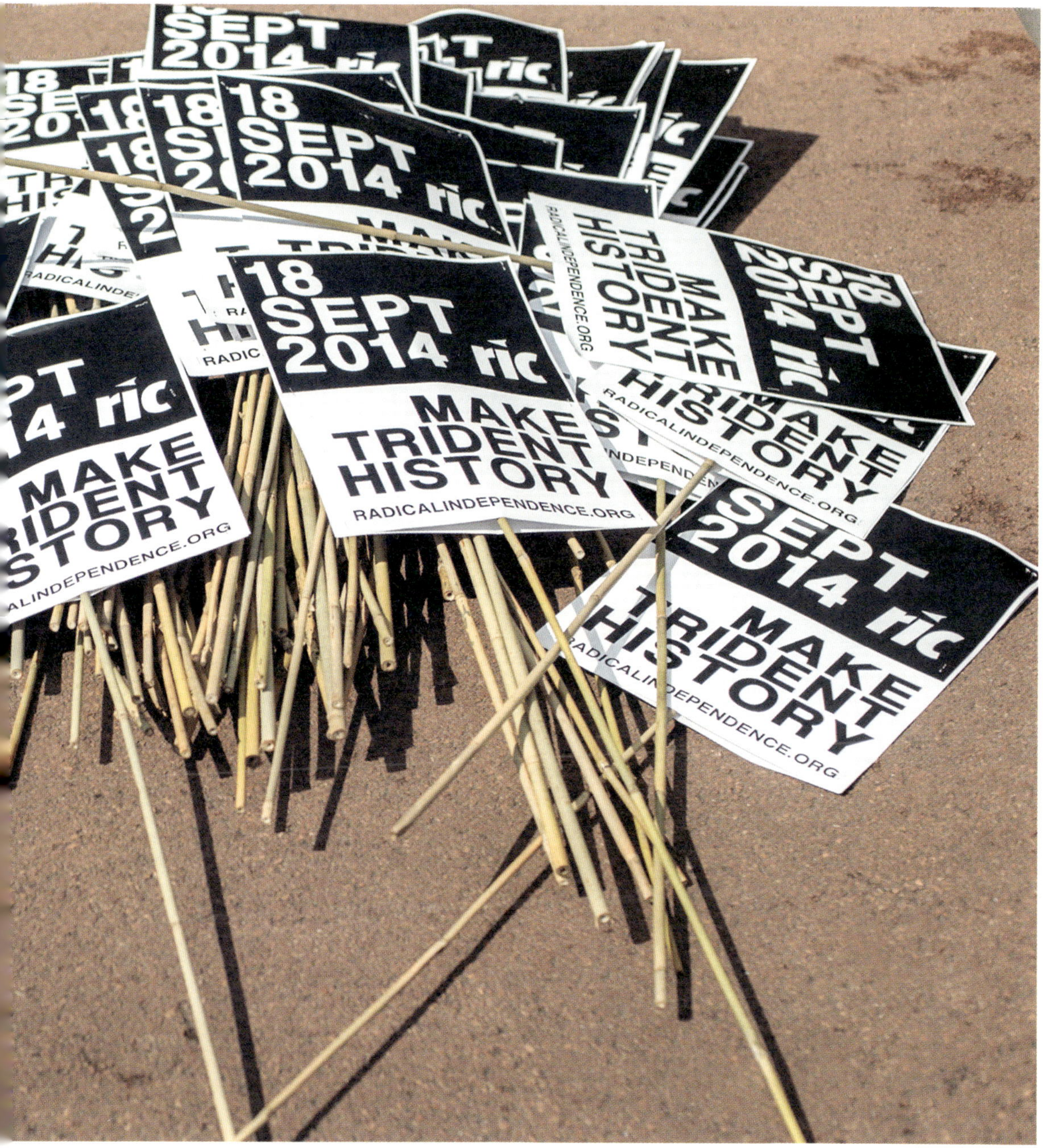
18 SEPT 2014 ric
MAKE TRIDENT HISTORY
RADICALINDEPENDENCE.ORG

Coorie (v)

An affectionate reference to cuddling, physical proximity. See also lumber.

In the frenzy of the campaign, a remarkably diverse group of people from all sorts of backgrounds put aside differences and worked closely in a spirit of camaraderie and shared spirit. What many people remember now was the warmth and coming-together of campaigning side by side — a renaissance in the meaning of community.

Is political community and shared feeling good for change or does it leave us in a bubble talking among ourselves?

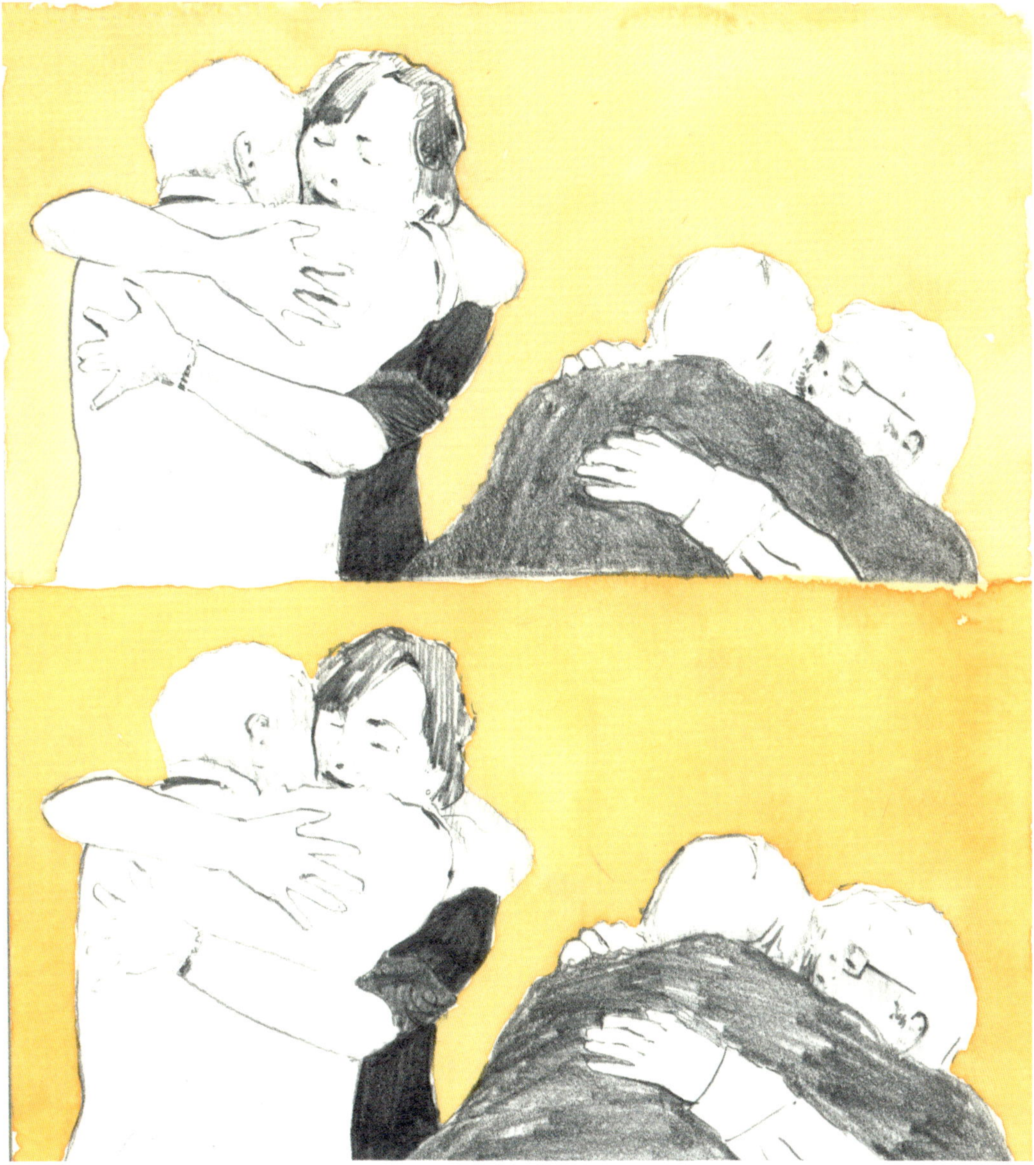

Coorie
Alistair Gow

Coorie

Dave Hook

Coorie is safe
And warm and restful
Close your eyes and coorie in

A wee coorie
Fuses strong and gentle
Sheltered in another skin

Resting overtired legs
A protective chest to lie your head
Arms length from the quarry's edge
Safe behind limbs and digits fence

You coorie when you're tired
Or in need of comfort
Or when your working day is done

A coorie is a deep breath
Inward, outward
Troubles from mind and air from lungs

A float releasing weight
A wrench releasing tension
A coorie doesn't debate
Or ask difficult questions

To coorie is to duck doon
Stoop
Bend
Crouch
Or kneel:
Behind a protector
Against the weather –
A human shield
When used in a sentence

It's the space between the lines
Either dig in for protection
Or make yirsel wee and hide

It's only a short step from coorie to coorin'
Tim'rous beastie –
Coorie in hen

We're aw in the same boat
Safety in numbers
Huddle together to stop from going under

Carried on a wave of camaraderie
Comrades, capitalists; democracy, anarchy

Except we don't have the same vision
Or share the same goals
When does a means to an end
Justify giving up core principles?

Beware of state controlled policies
Masquerading as support for those most
in need
Sometimes freedoms and equalities
Become the opposite of what they're
supposed to be

State guardianship – that sounds like a sort
of coorie
Appointed Protectors
A Governmental Coorie

From another angle that's state control
Coorying up to the status quo

So no –
The Independence Debate bore no resemblance to a coorie
It was exciting and scary and exhilarating
It was enlightening and frustrating
It was wildly emotional while trying to be completely rational
It was civic and national
It was nothing to do with ethnicity
It was finding common ground, talking, thinking and listening
It was linking arms with strangers like watching Rage Against The Machine in 1994 at T in the Park
It was really raging against the machine rather than playing a part
Fuck You I Won't Do What You Tell Me
Bairns not Bombs
If Not Now Then When?
Yes
But if it was one thing, it was active
It was exhausting and full of adrenaline
There was no place for a coorie in the referendum
The place and time for a coorie was the 19th of September

Haud on tight
It'll be awright
Coorie in noo then

Look at how far we've come
Hings'll never be the same again

Let's just take a moment to haud on to this feeling
Now's the time to rest your head

Then we'll get back up
And on with the business of what happens next

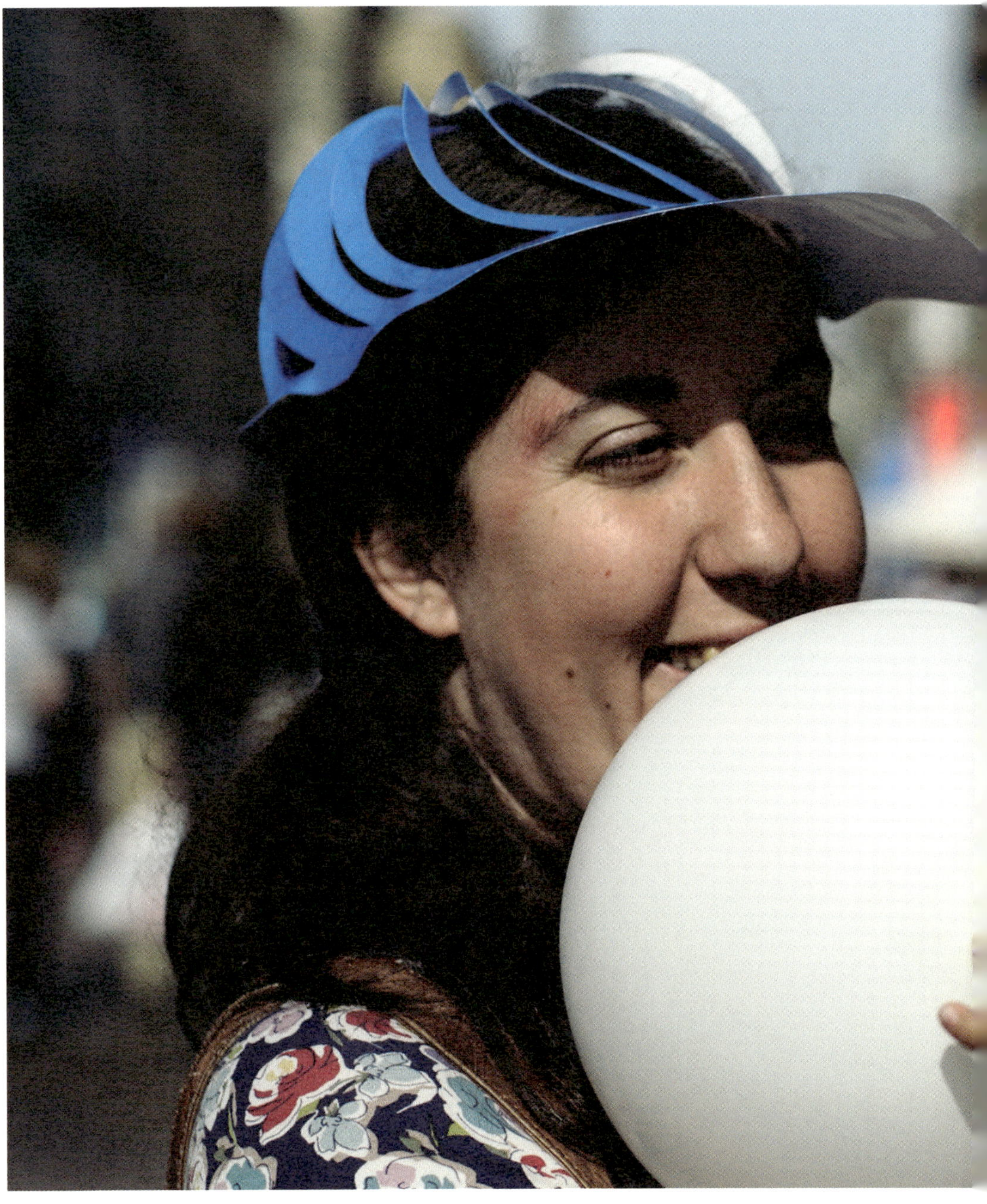

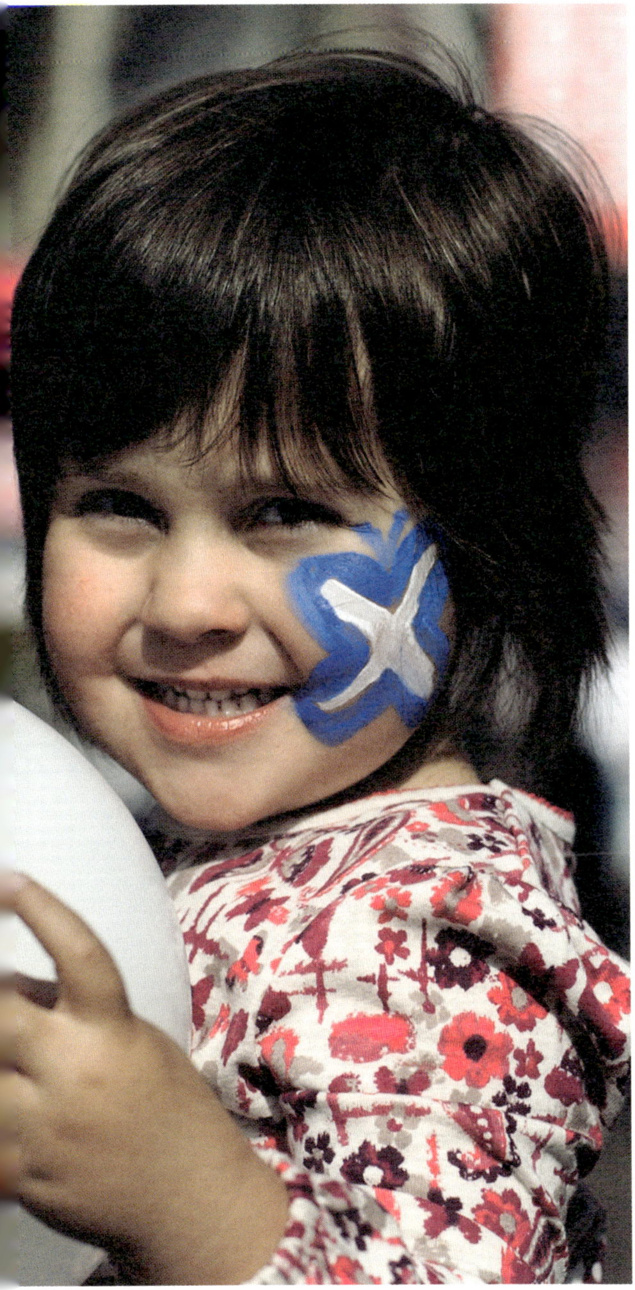

Our future is unknown. Good. Only in uncertainty can hope and possibility prosper. We choose the chance to fight for a better Scotland; we reject the offer to endure more of the same indefinitely. We are socialists, feminists, trade unionists, greens. We are from the peace movement, from anti-poverty campaigns, from anti-racists groups. We are community activists, civil liberty campaigners, the equalities movement and more.

RIC Declaration 2012

Beelin

In a state of extreme anger, resulting in vocal expressions of distaste and/or cursing. See also 'up to high dough'.

Many people in Scotland who are Unionists or suspicious of independence did not expect the size or strength of the Yes campaign and weren't ready for such a full-on assault on their beliefs. Scotland was certainly not an undivided nation.

How divided was Scotland? How much truth is there in claims of a nation fractured and bitter?

"This, then, gives us a hint of what Alex Salmond's brave new Scotland would really be like: a divided and rancorous society with a vindictive style of politics. If that sounds familiar, that's because it nicely sums up Scotland as it was before the Union."

Niall Ferguson

Extract from *Scottish referendum: Alone, Scotland will go back to being a failed state*

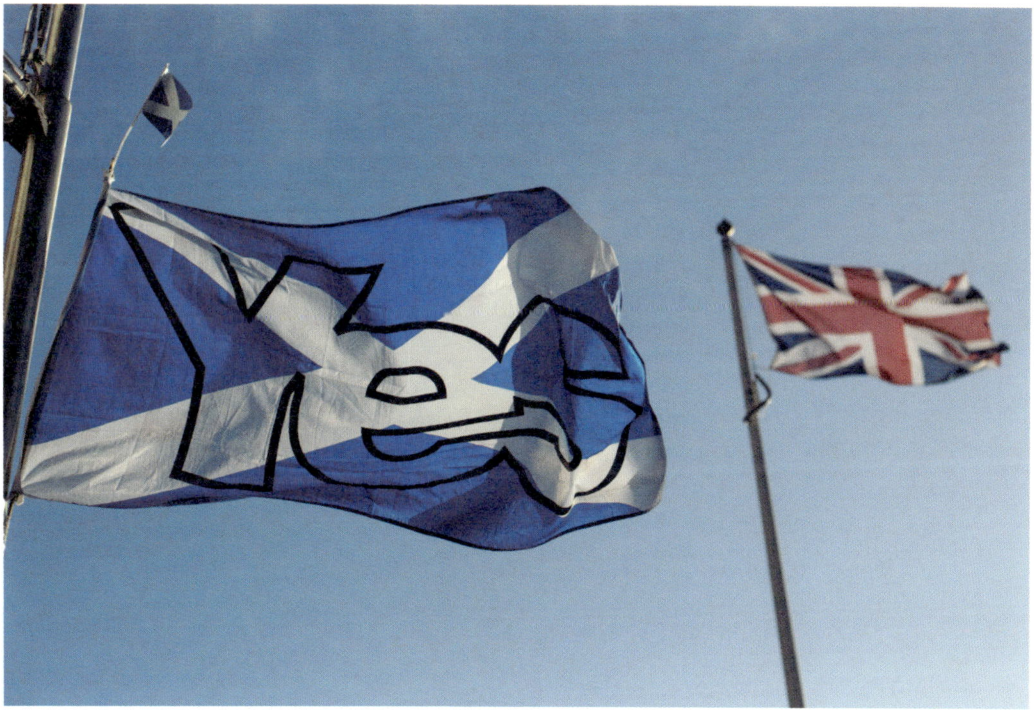

Peter McNally / Documenting Yes

This one time this mad cunt karate chopped a pigeon

Sam Small

The pigeon took off
people jumped aside
it was in the clear
then he rose
met it in the air
his turf now
eye to eye
beak to beak
karate chopped it
right in its sleekit cunt face

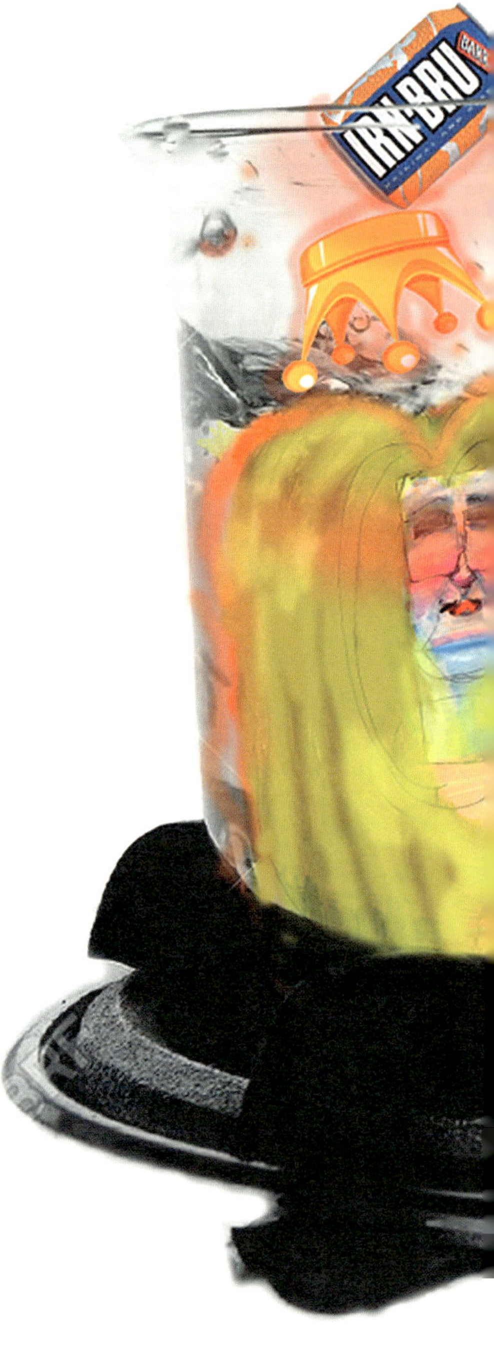

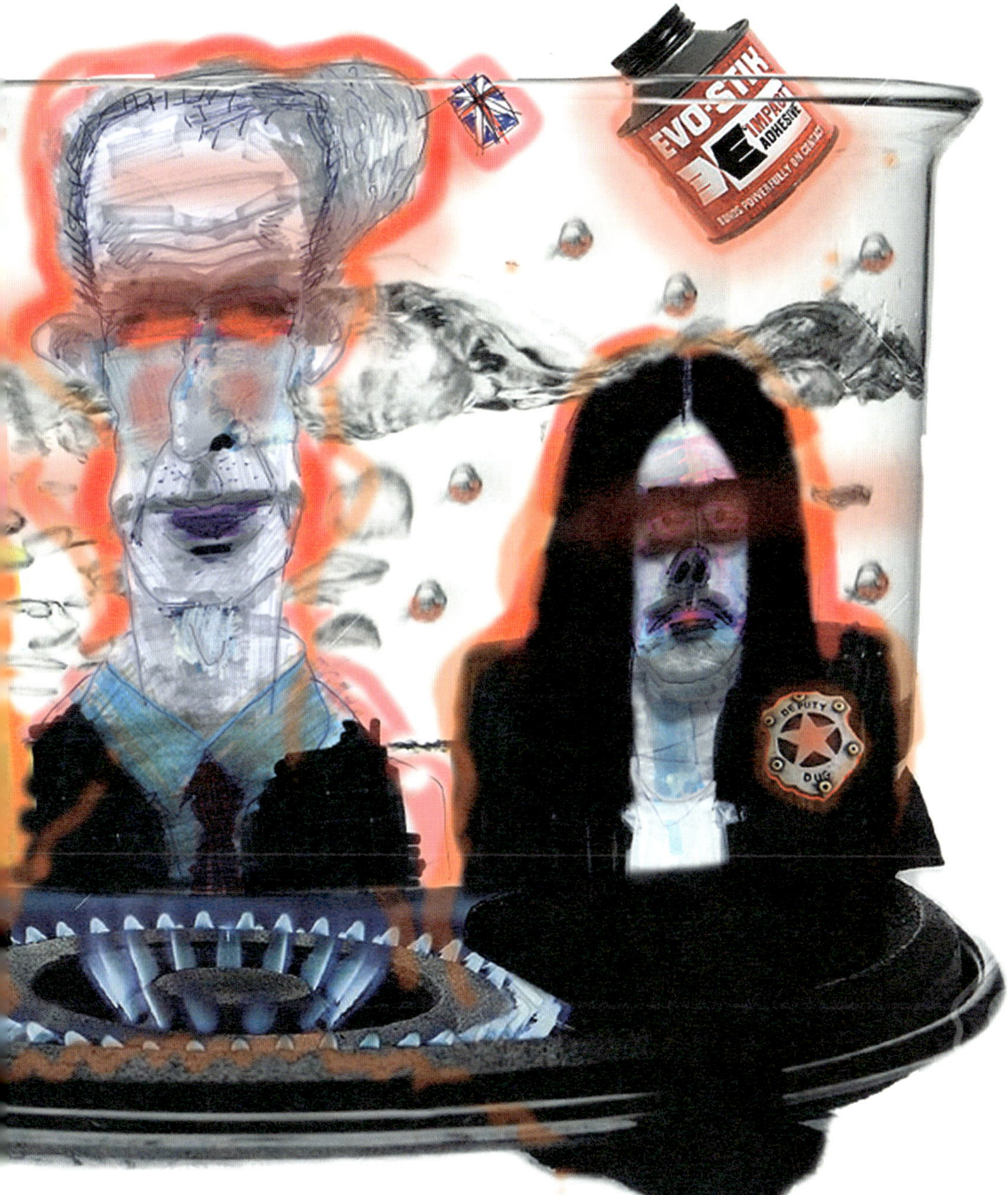

Beelin
Alasdair Strachen

Wheesht

Onomatopoeic command to be quiet, to hush.
'Hawd yer wheesht, man!"

To many it felt like as soon as more people wanted to think and talk and learn, more powerful groups wanted them to be quiet, stop talking and go back to doing as they were told — okay Scotland, back in your box.

Old media and old politics are seen by many to have failed Scotland. Is this perception fair? Were they as bad as many believe?

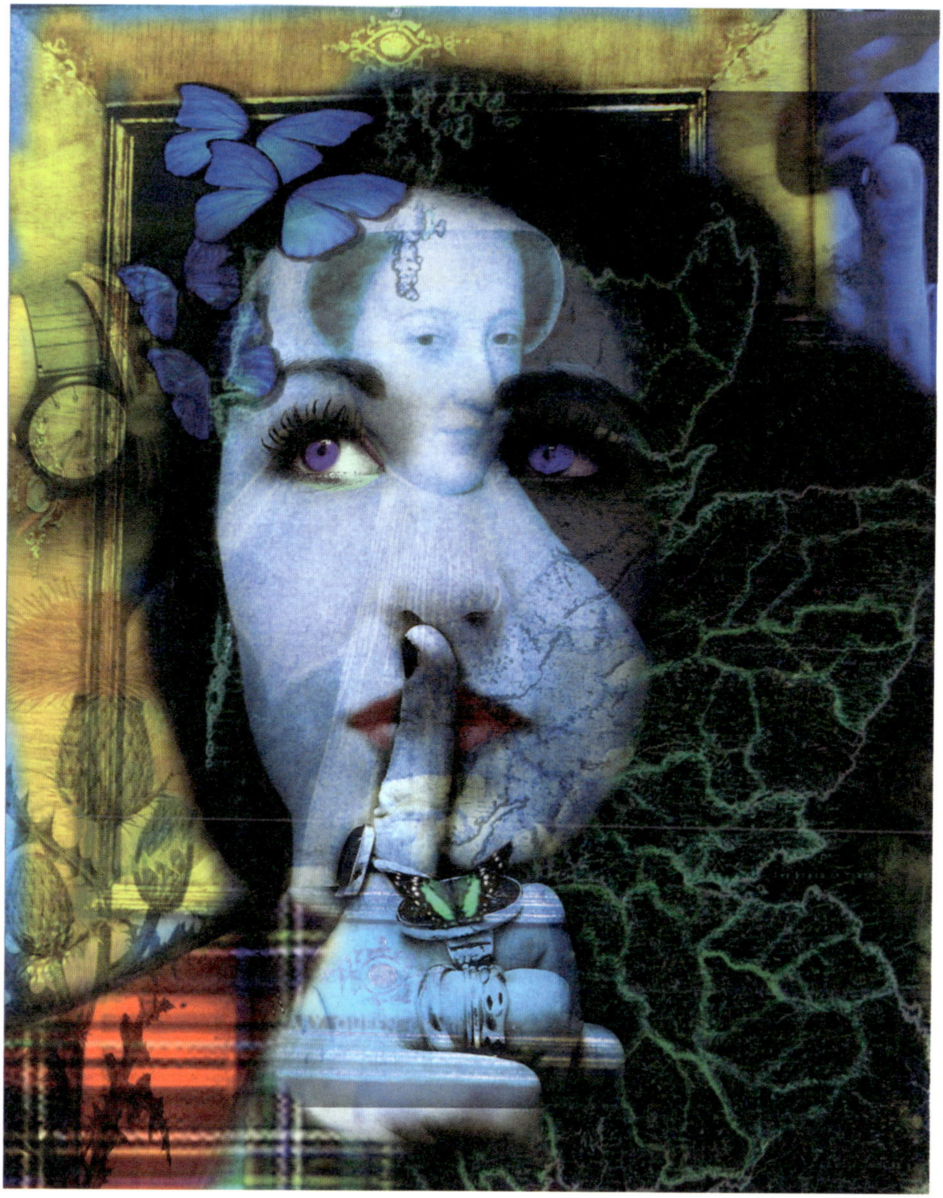

Wheesht
Ashley Cook

Wheesht

Janice Galloway

If liberty and equality are chiefly to be found in democracy, they will be best attained when all persons alike SHare in
government to the utmost. **Aristotle** Democracy must be something more than two wolves and a SHeep voting on what to
have for dinner. **James Bovard** WHEre justicE iS denied, wHere poverTy is enforced, where ignorance prevails,
and where any one class is made to feel that Society is an organized conspiracy to rob and degrade tHem, neither persons
nor property will be safe. **Frederick Douglass** None of this is necessary. There is no debt crisis. AuSterity is being used
as a Smokescreen to cover an ideologically - driven attack on the majority of tHe British public. **Jo Michell** If you see
oppreSSion of the poor, and justice and rigHteousness trampled in a country, do not be astounded. **King Solomon**
AuSterity is not part of tHe European treaties; democracy and the principle of popular sovereignty are. **Alexis Tsipras** The
ultimate trump card for the defenders of neoliberaliSm is THere Is No Alternative. **Robert W McChesney** Until the great
masS of the people SHall be filled with the sense of responsibility for each otHer's welfare, social justice can never be
attained. **Helen Keller** AlmoSt none of the huge amount of money loaned to Greece has actually gone there. It haS gone
to pay out private-Sector creditors... it's not about tHe money. It's about using deadlineS to force Greece to knuckle
under, to accept tHe unacceptable. **Dominic Stafford Uglow** In order to enSure the Survival of the ricHest, it is
democracy that has to be heavily regulated rather than capitalism. **Tari Ali** WHy is the Atlantic slowly filling with
crudE pEtroleum, thrEatening a millionS-of-years-old ecological balance? WHy did Traders at prominent
banks Take high-risk gambles with money enTrusted to Them ... leading to a global financial crisis that left millions
jobless? The belief in the supremacy of 'free' markets **George Monbiot** Justice cannot bE for onE Side alone
Eleanor Roosevelt

Policy makers abandoned the unemployed and turned to austerity because they Wanted to, not because tHEy had to **Paul Krugman** ThesE 'reformS' are tHreatening to the fuTure of the NHS ... our children Will look back and say how could you allow this to happen? **Dr Layla Jader** In Africa, in America, in Europe – protest arisEs not against dictatorships but against the shrEdding of democratic Systems: a narrow concentration of wealtH in a fraction of 1 percent of the population, stagnation for a large part of the resT, deregulation, and repeated financial crises, each one harsher than the last **Noam Chomsky** Both terrorists and governmentS make ordinary people pay for tHe actions of their governments. THe logic is the same **Arundhati Roy** The WealtH of the super-rich doEs not trickle down to improvE the economy, but tends to be amaSSed and sHeltered in tax havens with a negative effect on the Tax bases of the home economy **Tax Justice NeTwork**

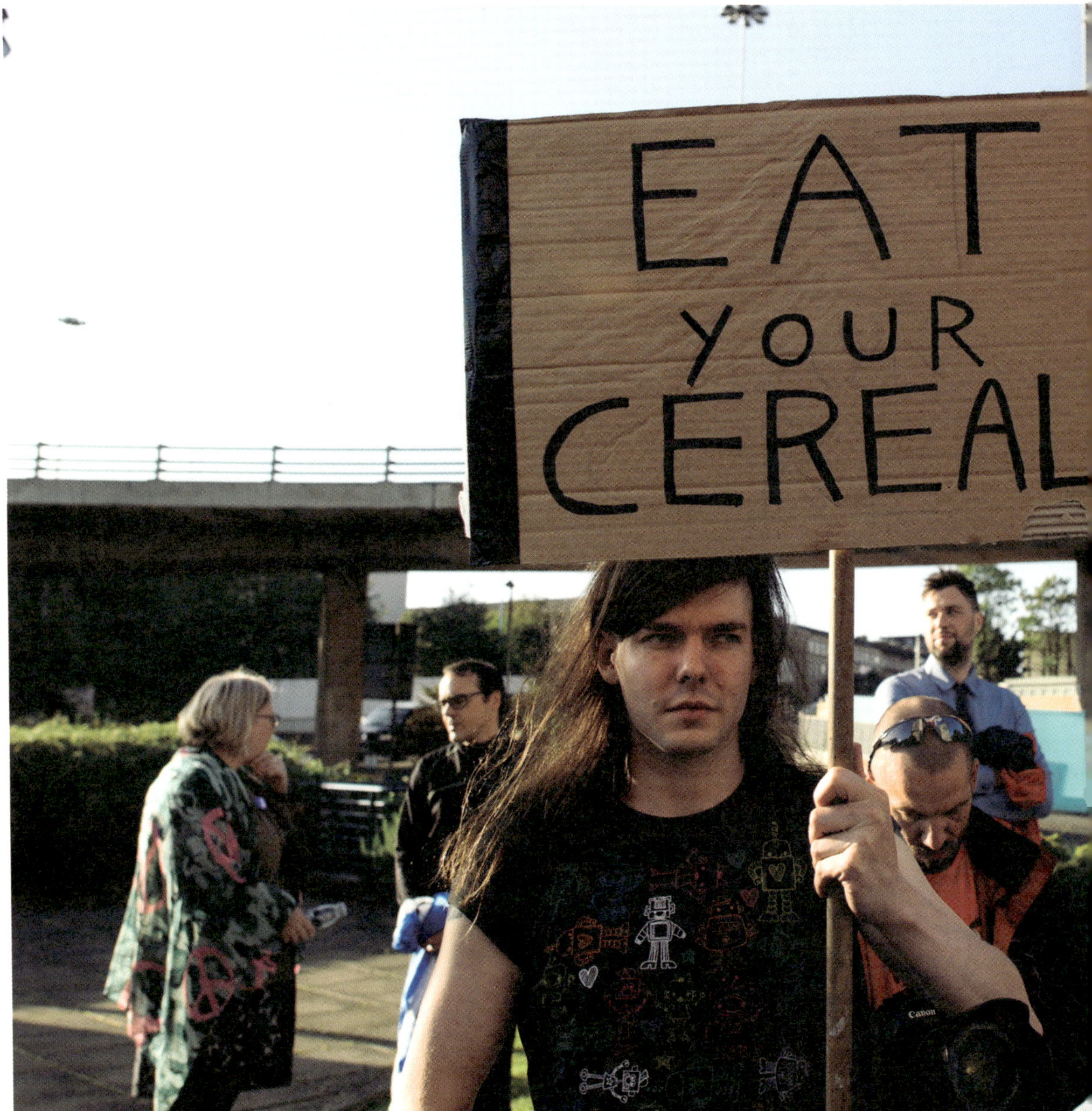

Peter McNally / Documenting Yes

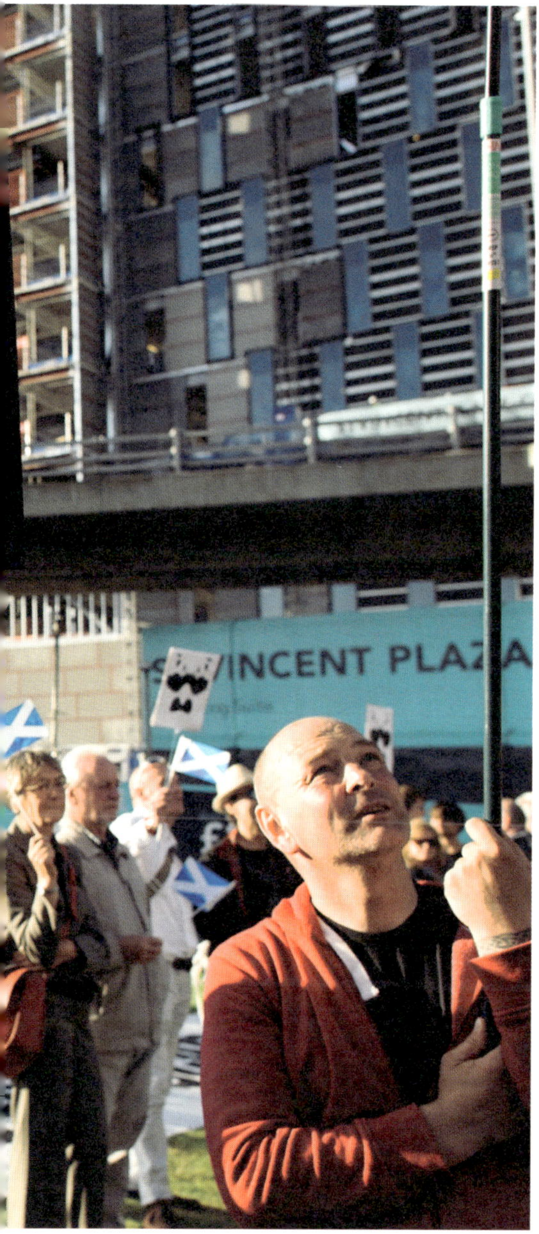

"Jenny [Hjul, Cochrane's wife and fellow columnist] said I should do what Darling asks. He's in charge after all. It's not really good journalism but what the hell does journalism matter? This is much more important."

Alan Cochrane

Extract from *Alex Salmond, My Part in His Downfall*

Swither (v)

To oscillate in determining the appropriate course of action.

People on both sides of the debate believe that they were the real winners – either because of the debate and its aftermath or the result and its outcomes. Scotland seems like a nation which has fundamentally failed to decide what it is.

How settled is Scotland's will? Are we two strong and opposed opinions living in one place – or is it more complicated?

Swither
June Carey

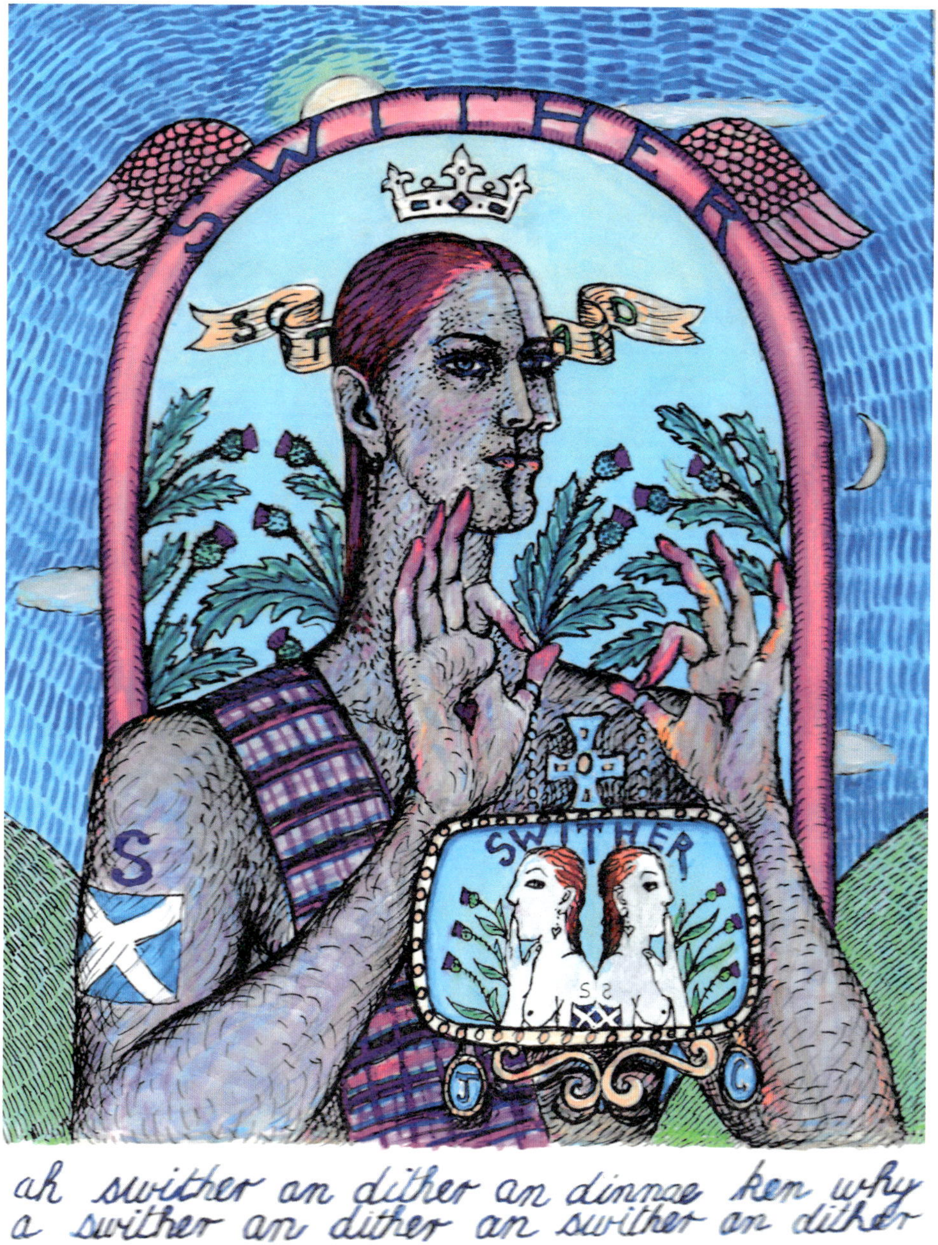
SWITHER
SWITHER
ah swither an dither an dinnae ken why
a swither an dither an swither an dither

Och, Scotland

Magi Gibson

Och, Scotland, ma wee cloven country,
sic a Jekyll 'n' Hyde o a nation,

one minute kneelin in piety prayin,
the next, howlin, whisky-raddled at the moon –

just like you to doff your *Hey Jimmy* bunnet
to the Queen, while bellowin

A Man's A Man for a' that,
we'll keep the red flag flyin' yet.

Always two sides to your story -
Heids – you're a country of limpid lochs and

heather-smothered mountains,
of kilts and haggises and sporrans.

Tails – you're a seethin', heavin' proletariat
in high-rise blocks and teemin' housin schemes.

You swing between your gothic nightmare fears
and sweet-as-Edinburgh-Rock soft-focus dreams.

But how you surprised the world, ma bonnie wee fechter,
when your disillusioned, dispirited masses, your

keep-your-heid-doon keep-your-joab-at-all-costs
workin classes

awoke
from their consumer-induced coma
arose
from their celebrity-besotted stupor

wrapped themselves in hope and Saltires
stuck their heads above the parapet of

this-is-how-it-is politics
dared to dream, to think of bringing into being

a different kind of Scotland, a different way of seeing.
Startled, the world turned its gaze

as whole crowds of Davids gathered
to sling a thousand chuckey-stanes

of why-the-fuck-shouldn't-we's,
of who-the-fuck-are-you-to-say-we-can't's

at the great galumphin Goliath
of global neo-liberal hegemony.

All of a sudden, wee Scotia, you were brave!
You were every ordinary man and every ordinary woman

in Catalonia and Quebec, in Chechnya and Kurdistan,
you were a glimpse of people-power possibility

of visionary, self-empowered democracy -
a triumph of sheer bloody-minded audacity -

a shaft of light to pierce the glowering clouds
of chained-to-the-markets global slavery.

But just as quick as you grew bold,
so too you grew afraid

when those whose power you dared to challenge
rattled their sabres, made ever-fiercer threats

and in the final count, you displayed the split
that always haunts your psyche -

deep as the ancient Caledonian fault
that cleaves the very rock that forms you.

"Caught between the reassuring solidity of 'now' and the indefinite promise of 'soon', many Scots rejected change in 2014. That does not mean they didn't want change. Far from it. So the task at hand is to make that future more solid by beginning to make the change real. When the people of Scotland are next asked to hope for a better Scotland, it is not enough that they can close their eyes and imagine it.

They must have seen it being born all around them, where they live and where they work. The moment when Scotland can take some time to gaze into the future has passed – for now. The moment when we must roll up our sleeves and begin the work of building is upon us."

Extract from *Common Weal book of policy proposals for the 2016 Scottish elections*, forthcoming

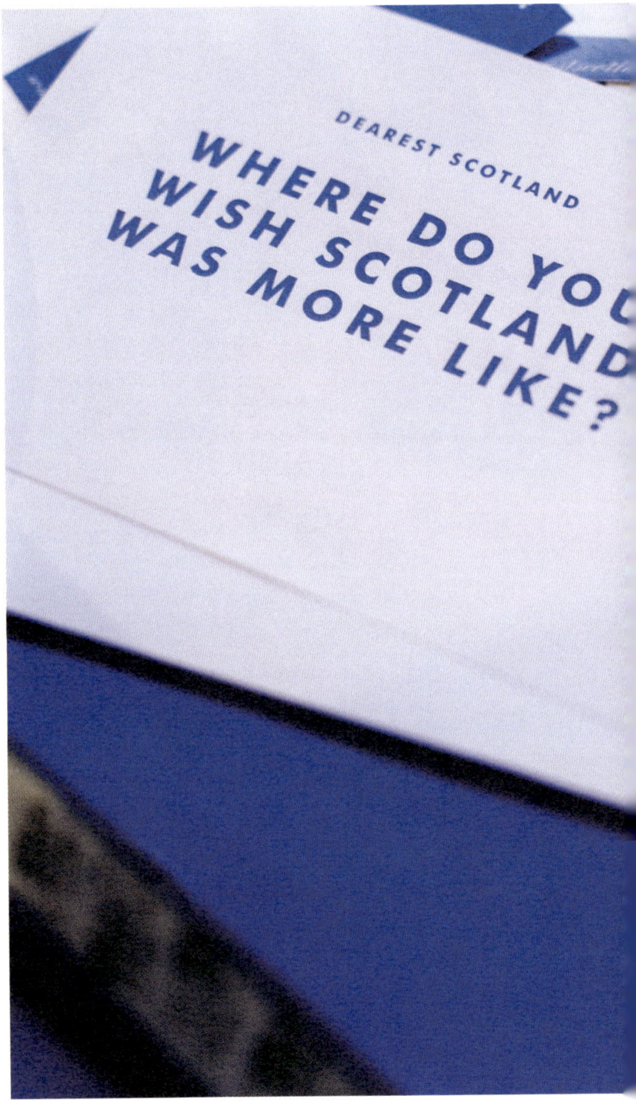
DEAREST SCOTLAND
WHERE DO YO
WISH SCOTLAN
WAS MORE LIKE?

Peter McNally / Documenting Yes

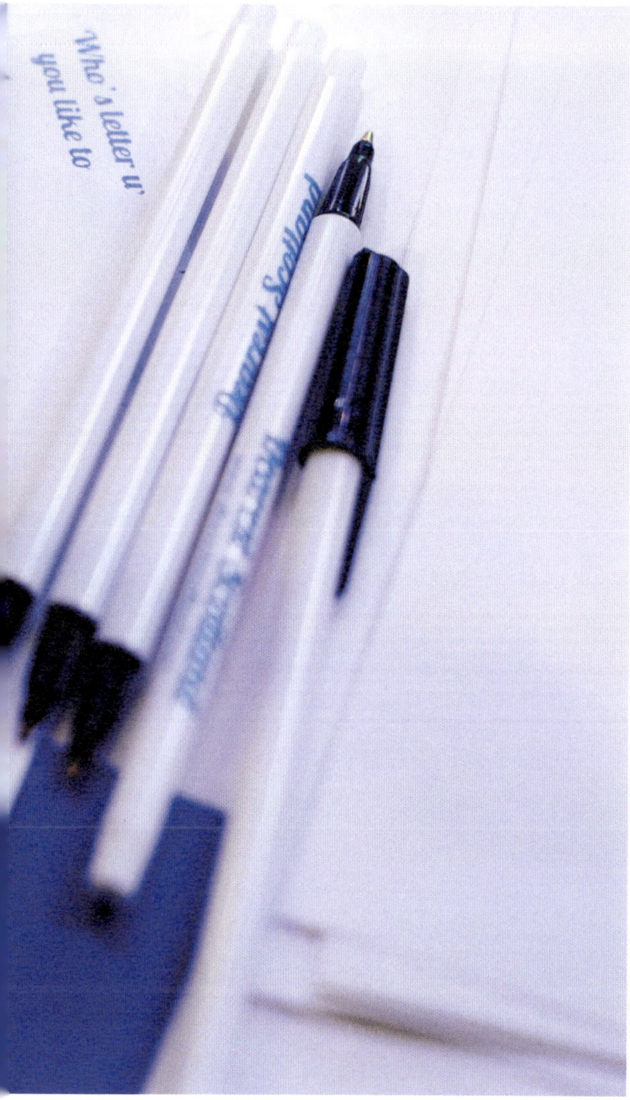

When you realise you're in a relationship in which the two of you want different things, where your hopes and dreams are taking you in different directions, you don't hesitate because you're not sure what you're going to get in the divorce settlement; you make the decision and then you sort things out afterwards."

Val McDermid

Extract from *Scottish writers on the referendum – independence day?*

Dreich

An iconic diagnosis for Scottish weather, epitomising the classic characteristics of an overcast, rainy, cold and generally intolerable day.

On 19 September 2014, Scotland woke up to the realisation that it was over – the grassroots campaign, the big thinking, the hopes of many. It was a grey and sombre day. Was it the end?

How did the new, awakened radical Scotland deal with defeat?

"We lost. Get over it. Every second we spend licking our wounds is a second we lose for the fight. And fight we must. And fight we will. We made much of this land our Scotland, not theirs. So now we hold our territory. Then we take theirs. Wipe your eyes. On your feet. Grab your stuff. Let's get started."

Robin McAlpine

Extract from *Wipe your eyes. On your feet.*

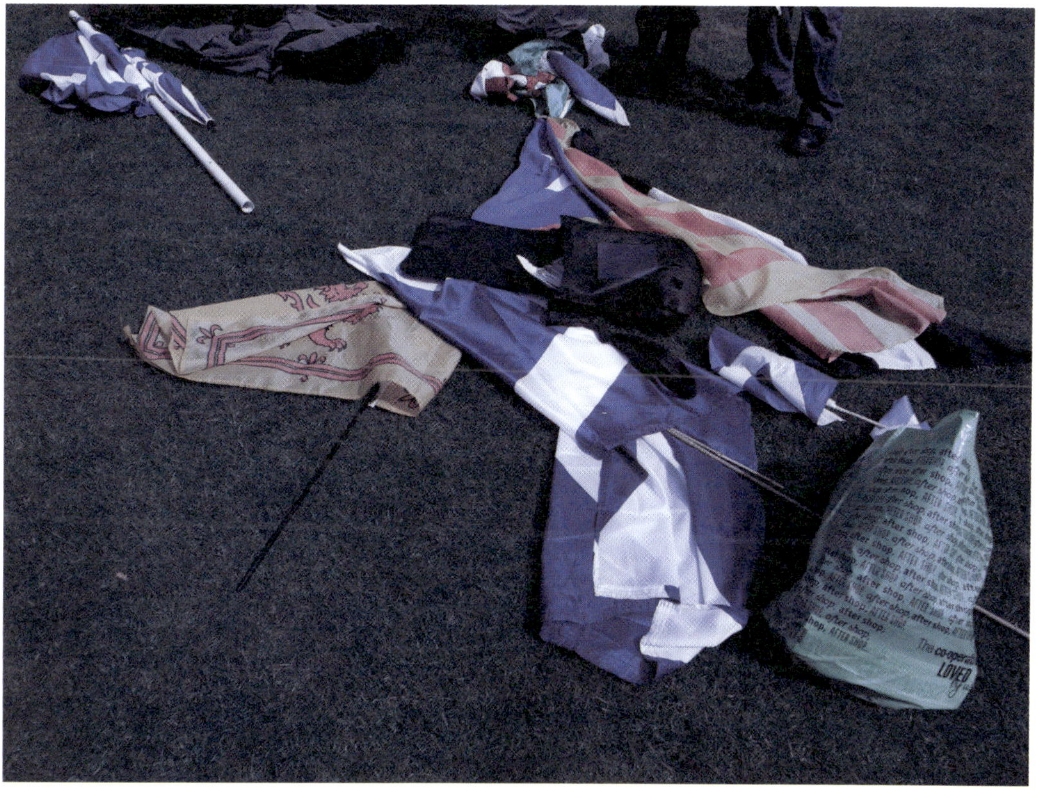

Peter McNally / Documenting Yes

Dreich

Ian Dunn

Scotland lives in the dreich.

We grow up in endless grey, wet Sunday afternoons with our noses pressed against windows, looking at weather that isn't even horrible enough to be exciting.

Then we spend our adult lives,
awaking in darkness and trudging out of the house into the damp and the cold.

And when we die, it's only fitting if we're buried in miserable weather,
raindrops mingling with the mourner's tears.

Scottish winters are six months of dreich,
wet grey misery weighing on us,
forcing us down to crawl along the pavements.

When we talk about the character of a people,
the nature of a culture,
the weather is rarely mentioned. It's all history,
art, politics and hopes,
but we live in the weather.

It's with us every moment of the day,
and who we are, how we are,
is a dreich people.

Grounded by generations of looking out at endless grey cloud,
it forms us more than anything save family.

Our literature is stories of the cynical and rain soaked.
Our films are portraits of grotty lives lived beneath overcast skies.
That's not to say Scottish culture is one of misery and fear,
but we cannot ignore that grey is ever-present in the palate of our lives.

On September 19th last year I was driving from Stirling to Glasgow in the early afternoon,
the sky had greyed, the rain was falling, and the traffic was jammed.

Scotland has rarely looked dreicher.
Grey skies, grey moods.
The future stretched out like an endless Scottish winter.

The months since, with their endless 'he said, she said' political spats,
have rarely given the impression that a brighter day is coming.
Yet it's amazing what you can find in language.

The word Dreich itself comes from the Middle English, where it meant long suffering.
Easy enough to see how it morphed into a description of the Scottish weather.
That evolved from the Norse word *drjúgr*,
meaning 'enduring, lasting'.

Grey is not just the colour of looming,
spitting clouds,
It's the colour of stone and steel;
things that last.

Scottishness lasts.

300 years in a Union with a much bigger, more powerful neighbour,
and Scottish identity has rarely been stronger.

That endurance comes from the dreich,
from walking through the rain, and the cold,
and the wind.
It makes us strong and with strength
comes hope.

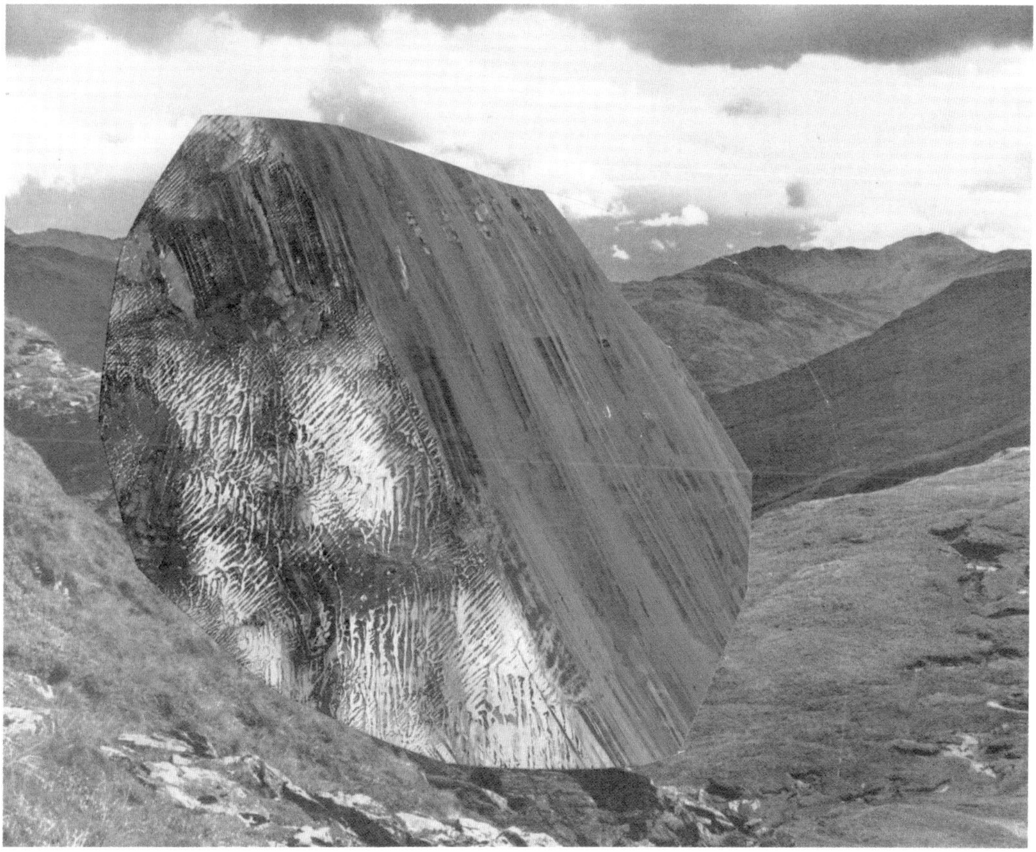

Driech
Rachel Mimiec

Feart

Timorous, intimidated, or just plain petrified.

Despite all the rammy and stooshie, the gabbin and gallusness, Scotland said no. Were we just too afraid to say yes? Or was it something else?

In the end, what made Scotland vote no? Fear? Belief? Not being ready? Not being convinced?

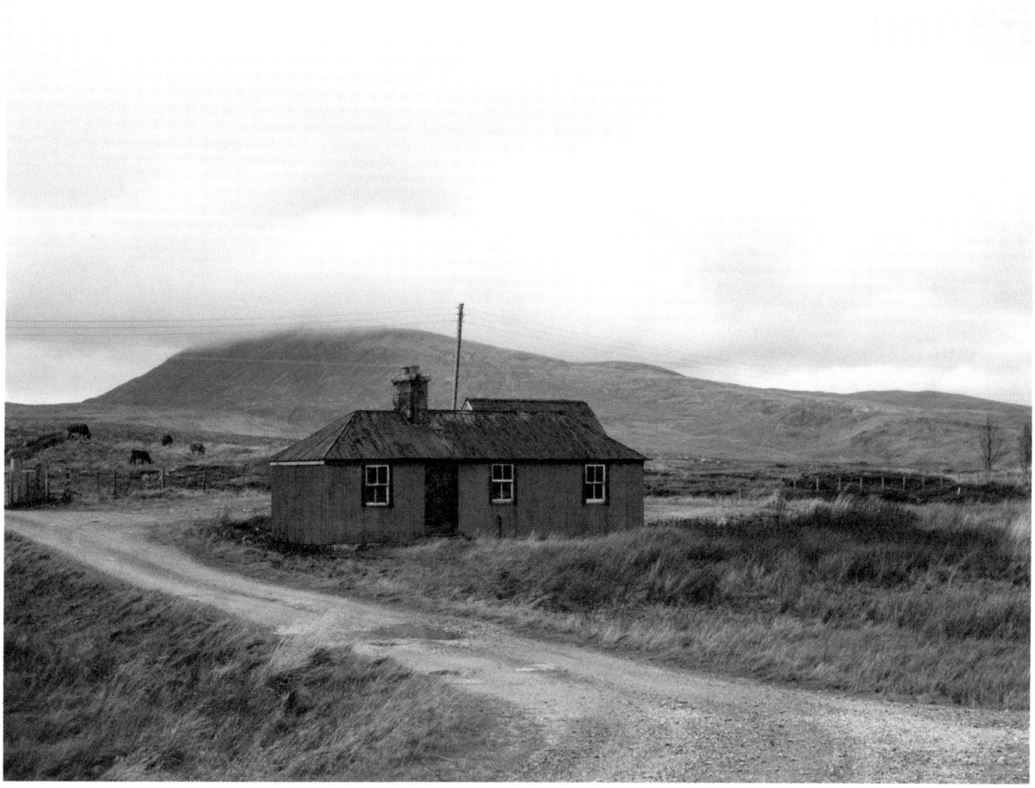

Peter McNally

Feart

Aileen McKay

When I was wee I was scared of the dark. My parents installed a nightlight, its soft glow filling the corner of my bedroom to chase the shadows away. I could see what had been out of sight before. I could see that there were no monsters hiding under my bed, concealed in the pile of clothes on my chair, or hidden behind my bookshelf.

Without wishing draw a heavy-handed analogy between knowledge and light, it is true to say that when a light shines, shadows disappear: murkiness gives way to clarity. Put simply, things become clearer. The more you know about something the less scary it becomes, the more manageable it seems, and the more you feel in control — no, the more you *are* in control.

However, when we're afraid, our brain shuts down; reasoning stops and we short-circuit to emotional responses. Monsters crawl back to take up residence under our beds and the unknown becomes terrifying. Since our referendum we have accused each other of being afraid, too feart of our own independence.

But I don't think it was that. In our own lives we strive for independence from an early age. Being able to leave home, pay our own bills, or choose when we go to bed are all forms of independence, ways of leaving dependency behind. Aye, that's not to say that this doesn't come with its own challenges and pitfalls — and it's not to say that all of those things are easy all of the time. But would you ever go back to how you lived as a child now? Would you let someone else take charge? Sure, it might be hard, but those challenges are completely attached to your sense of selfhood, because making those decisions — both big and small — that affect your life is what makes you you. So independence is a natural state of being.

I think what we were actually afraid of was *setting out* towards our independence. And of what ugly truths about ourselves we might discover on the way. I'm thinking of the radio silence around Scotland's very active role in the atrocities of the British Empire, especially on the school syllabus and the disgustingly euphemistic exhibition of 'curios' in our National Museum.

The first steps into the Great Unknown are always the hardest. But here's the thing: we have already taken those first steps.

Over the last few years, huge swathes of a population who had never before had reason to care about Politics (with a capital P) started to engage. Beyond the silly sniping and costly game-playing of UK party politics, Scotland's citizens were asking questions...

How do we write a constitution that enshrines human rights for all of our people?

What makes a just taxation structure and how can we build one?

How do we help our society's weakest in a sustainable and dignified way?

And we started to come up with answers.

To borrow from Alan Bissett's Fringe show from this time last year, *The Pure, the Dead, and the Brilliant*:

'It wis time.
Ye were awake.
The lights were gaun on.
How could ye unlearn what ye had learned?'

And that's just it: we have learned, we have switched the lights on, and – I hope – chased away the shadows, to see that there is nothing truly worth being afraid of in the prospect our independence. Nervous? Maybe. A wee bit worried? Perhaps. But feart? Not a chance.

As I write now – the news headlines editing away the Troika's attack on the Greek people and our own government's attack on us – we have our task cut out for us, and the stakes are higher than we could know. We must work as if we live in the early days of a better world. And in that labour there is no place for fear.

"We want a Scotland that is equal for all genders. But we can't achieve that without confronting the current relations of power in our society that privilege white, straight, rich men.

The question we want to answer is not whether Scotland should be an independent country, but how a yes vote can change the lives of Scottish women....We don't want to see a post-Yes Scottish society that's simply more of the same- because Britain is typical of neo-liberal neo-patriarchy: it is an archaic and masculine state. Britain is inseparable from its neoliberal institutions, which have systematically shattered and dismantled any sense of collective struggle for women's equality. Britain has duped women into thinking they've won some concessions for equality, but it has in reality set us back.

Breaking up Britain can help stop this trajectory, and it opens up a tiny crack for new struggles to ferment, and for new radical victories. If the official Yes campaign fails, it's because of its gender blindness: that they've failed to show how a Yes vote can transform the current consensus which creates and recreates inequality for women."

Cat Boyd and Jenny Morrison

Extract from *Scottish Independence – A Feminist Response*

Feart
Anderston Torp

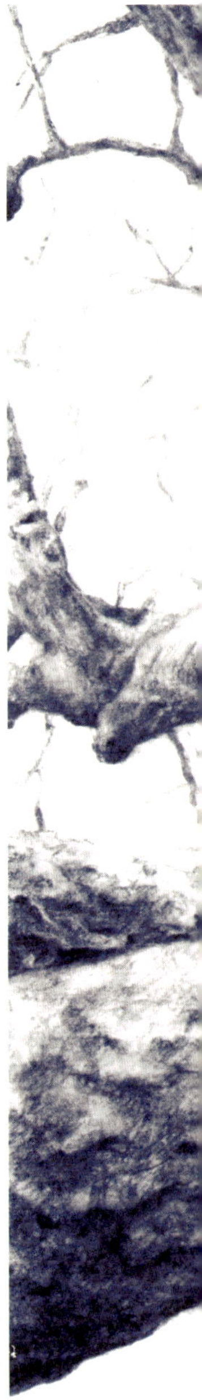

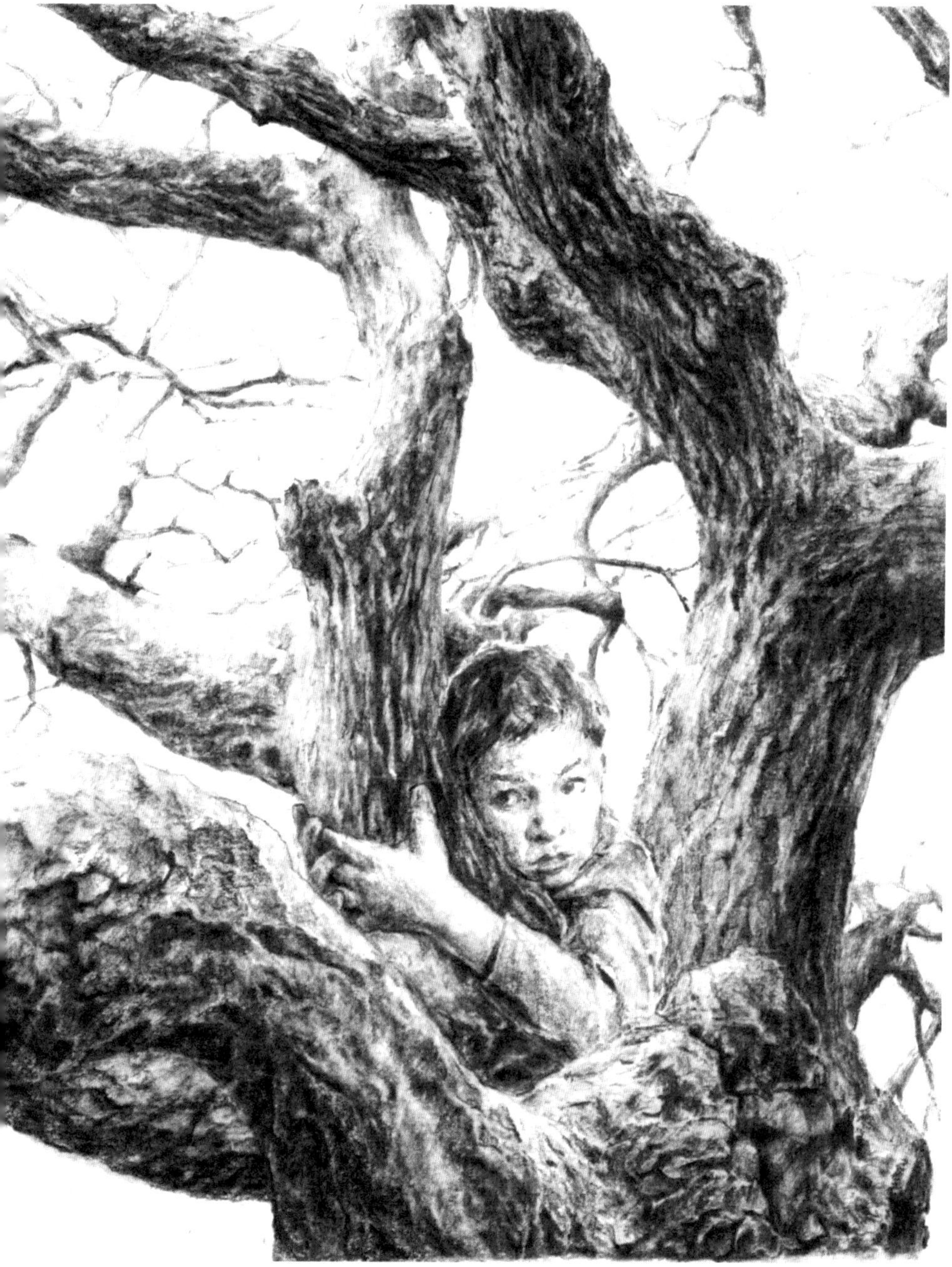

Thrawn

**A determined, stubborn, recalcitrant demeanour.
See also: bam, radge, gallus.**

Despite the crushing defeat, within days the Yes movement was back on its feet and fighting again. Campaigners have shown a genuinely surprising unwillingness to 'stay down'.

Independence supporters and many observers now believe independence is a matter of time.
Are they right?

"...with the younger generations strongly weighted on the Yes side while the over 50s stuck with caution, the stage is set for the politics of change in Scotland. If the intention of the referendum was to close down radical debate about Scotland's future, then it has been a signal failure, more of a starting gun than a finish line defeat."

Donald Smith

Extract from *Scotland's Democracy Trail*

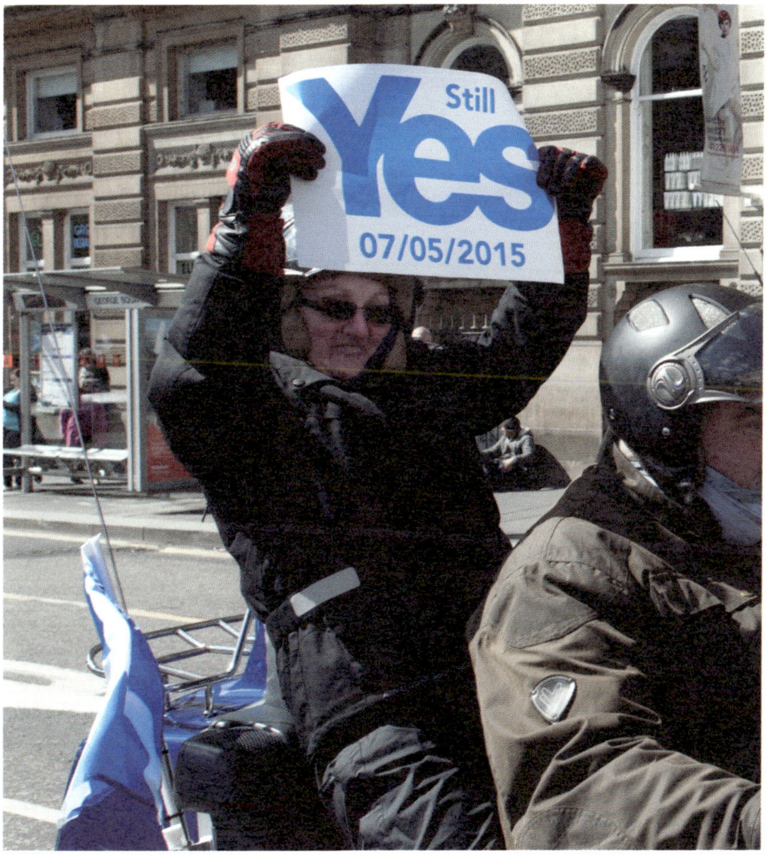

Peter McNally / Documenting Yes

Thrawn
David Greig

I knew we'd lost after Clackmannan. I went to bed not long after that. Lucie stayed up with the lap-top watching the other results come in. I slept fitfully. Every now and then I'd mumble... 'anything new?' and Lucie would say 'No.' Sometime around 9am I got up and made coffee. I had no appetite.

I drank my coffee and looked out at the dank of the morning. The Forth was grey, the sky was grey, a soft mist hung in the air... I felt as if I'd awoken from a dream: as if the last two years had all been part of a fitful night of colour and possibility and madness and now this... this was the hangover, this was the dawn. I felt foolish and a little ashamed. 'How could I ever have thought the world was other than this. This is real. This is life. This is who you are.'

Lucie said we should go for a walk. Both of us had taken the friday off work in the hope, I suppose, of sleeping off a night of celebration. Now we just wanted to get away from everything.

We got in the car. I didn't know where we would go. We didn't really care. In the end we followed the Forth up to Culross where there were woods and walks I knew from running. As we drove I put on my ipod and a song came up which had been a private indyref anthem for me... Stay Gold by First Aid Kit.

'The sun shone high those few summer days,
left us in a soft wide eyed haze,
it shone like gold,
it shone like gold.
But just as the moon it shall stray,
so the dawn goes down today
no gold can can stay,
no gold can stay.'

Scotland at the summer's end is green and lush and wet. The roadside verges hang with brambles and elderberries. The woods are an endless deep green. We drove along the road to Kincardine heavy with the sense of summer's going. The first aid kit song has a lovely, plaintive chorus...

'What if our hard work ends in despair,
what if the road don't go anywhere,
oh I wish it could Stay Gold.'

In the fields by the roadside, cylindered hay bales lay scattered over the stubble like dropped pills. Amongst them three ancient stones stood in a circle. The farmer had carefully drawn his harvester around them: an island of the deepest past. A reminder that there were people here before there was a Scotland and, I suppose, there will be people here long after.

We drove down the hill, past the ruins of Culross abbey. and into the village along the cobbled lane. Culross was built on coal but unlike the other mining villages of the Fife coast Culross's wealth was pre-industrial revolution. Its houses are a glimpse of a Scotland which knew nothing other than being wholly itself; a kingdom from where ships and merchants sailed out of the Forth to trade with Scandanavia and Holland.

We parked and walked a little way along the old railway line towards the giant brutalist cubes of Longannet power station and, across the river, the towers and smoke of Grangemouth. When I was growing up I was taken on school trips to gaze in awe at these twin cathedrals of the future. Longanett and Grangemouth were symbols of Ladybird book modernity: a socialist Scotland where clever Scottish men were shaping the world and solving its problems, while bright Scottish women hung clean washing in front of the sparkling gables of new council houses as Scottish children played, healthy and clean, on municipal greens.

The railway line's a coastal path now, the Valleyfield pits a park.

We turned up a hillside into some woods. We hadn't spoken much. I said maybe we had to live up to our ideals. We had to 'work harder'. I said, maybe I would finally set up that Commonweal Running Club I'd talked about... getting kids from deprived areas into running... On the running vest we'd have the slogan... 'all of us first.' I was burbling, really. We walked on following whatever paths happened to open up to us. Willing ourselves to get lost.

I noticed Lucie was crying.

Finally we came to a sign which pointed down a puddled lane: 'To The Plague Graves'. We laughed. What better way to cheer ourselves up. We set off down the lane just as a soft drizzle started to fall.

That was when Lucie spoke. She said she didn't feel sad, she felt embarrassed. She felt embarrassed for Scotland. The fear and intimidation of the last weeks of the campaign, the desperate pleas and the offers... it had been all been so transparent to her and she had felt so sure Scotland would see through them. Her idea of Scotland, she said, was of a strong, thrawn country: a country that would stand up for itself and forge its own way in the world. But in the fitful sleepless night she had watched it capitulate, meekly, willingly in it's own submission. Her tears, she said, weren't sadness but shame.

I wasn't crying and I wondered why. I had put two years into the referendum. I would have been entitled to some grief. But I realised that I too didn't feel sad. What I felt was worse than sad, it was relief; the sort of relief you feel when you fail to get a new job, or your team are beaten in the final, or all the tickets of your lottery come up except the last...Relief. The relief of knowing that everything is back to normal.

When everything is back to normal you don't need to change your idea of yourself. You don't need to take responsibility. You don't need to think new thoughts. You don't need to forge new relationships. You can go back to being the way you've always been. Deep personal change is fun to dream about but close up, it's frightening. Failing to change can feel heroic, especially you did your best after all. Now, in guilt-less failure, you can go back to the easy comfort of complaining and shrugging and saying 'I told you so' and dreaming about what might have been.

The lane had narrowed to a path and the path was now narrowing to a trod through an old plantation woodland. Like all plantation woodland it was a spooky, dark green place, half nature, half architecture. We followed the trod through blueberry bushes into the deep of the wood until we came to a small clearing.

In the clearing was a stone ruin of a small house. Amongst the moss and the wet black stones there was a plaque. The plaque said that here a whole family, including seven children, had died of plague. Beside the plaque were some old plastic flowers.

Lucie and I stood and looked at the scene. It seemed both poignant, and at the same time, utterly meaningless. We sat on some stones.

And then it came to me, a sudden wave of feeling, an upthrust not of grief but something else – refusal, like a horse at a jump. 'I refuse,' I thought. 'I refuse to go back to normal. I refuse to let the last two years be a dream. I refuse the proposition that this is over. I am changed. We are changed. We made that change ourselves and I refuse to go back to how it was before. We will continue to make ourselves anew.'

We walked back out through the blueberries and bracken, to the mud of the lane.
The drizzle had lifted a little.

Lucie took my hand and squeezed it.

Thrawn.

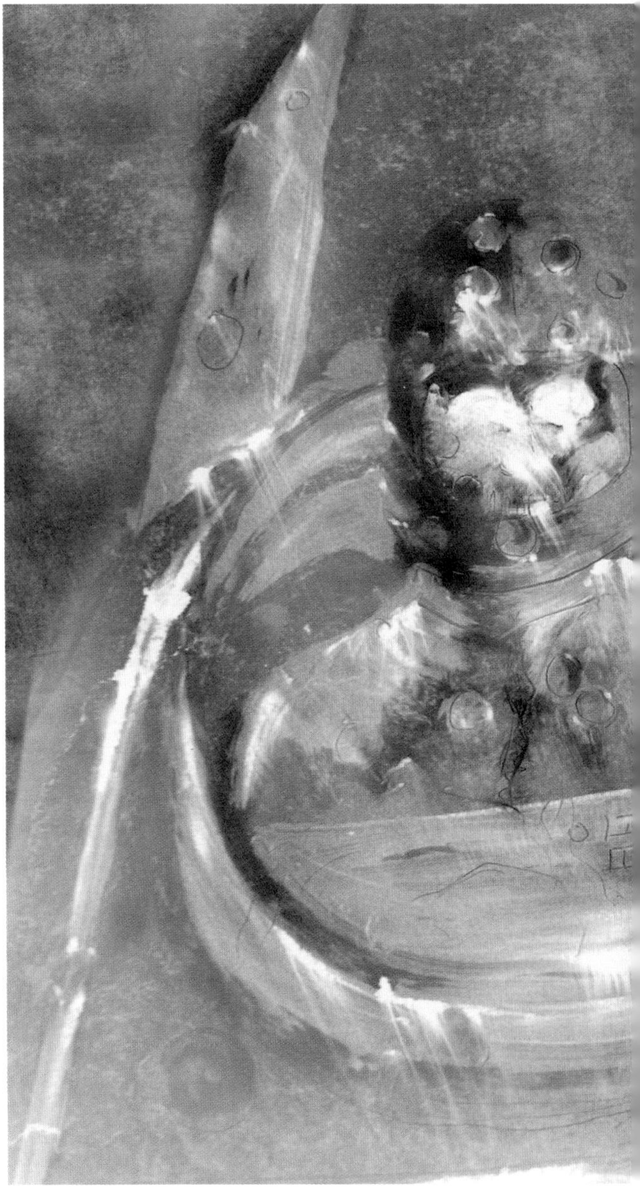

Thrawn
Duncan McGillvray

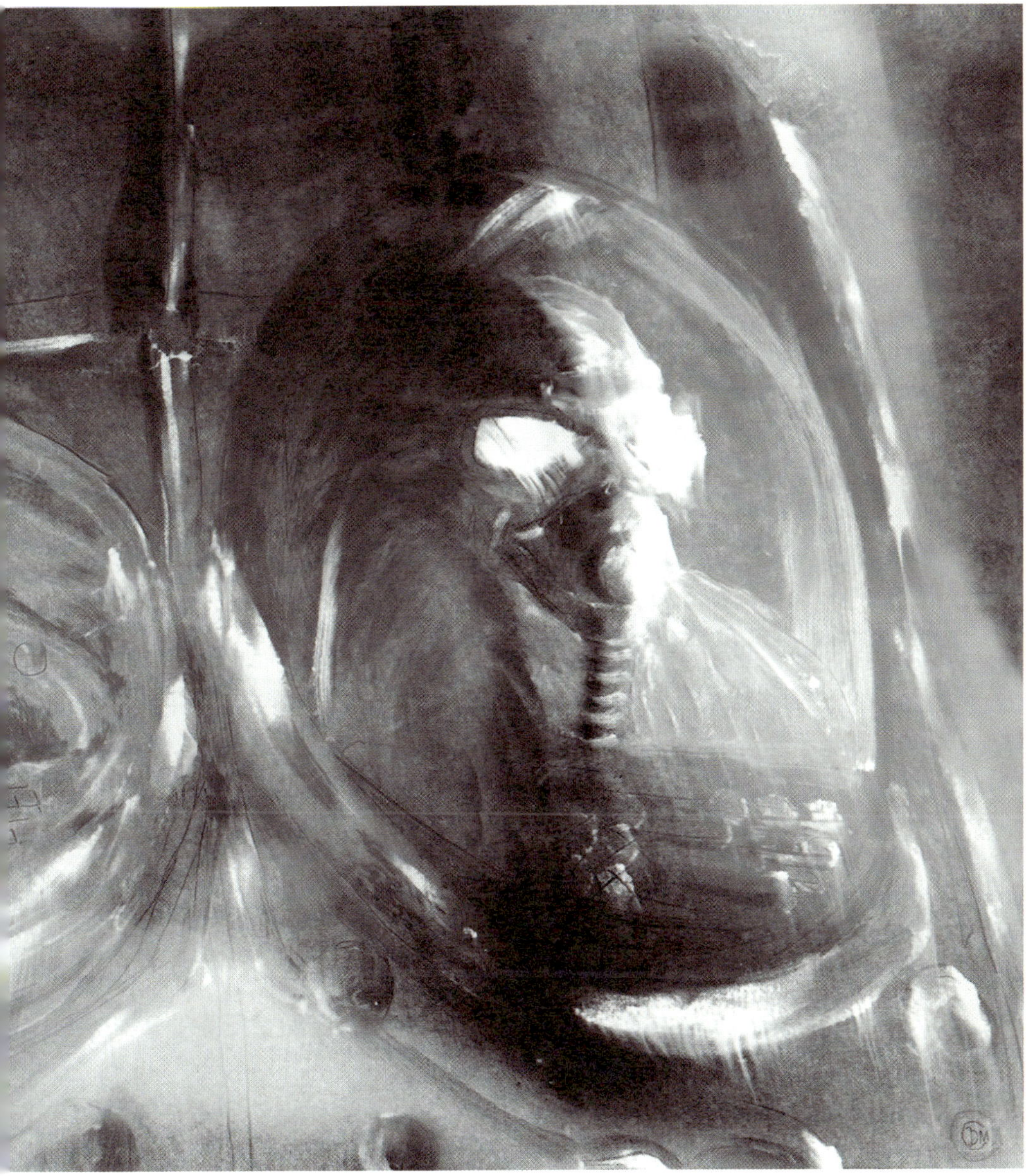

Mind (v)

To remember, recall, recollect past experiences.
"Mind that yon time Scotland voted naw?"

Time passes. Both the excitement and enthusiasm – and the pain – drift further into the past. The campaign will live on in history books and in the memory. But what will these pages and these memories say about us?

What is left from the campaign? What should we take from it? What should we dispose of?

"Pessimists will say there is now nothing left in
Scotland for Home Rule to improve.
I deny that, if we work as if in the early days
of a better nation."

Alasdair Gray

Extract from *Work as if you live in the early days of a better nation*

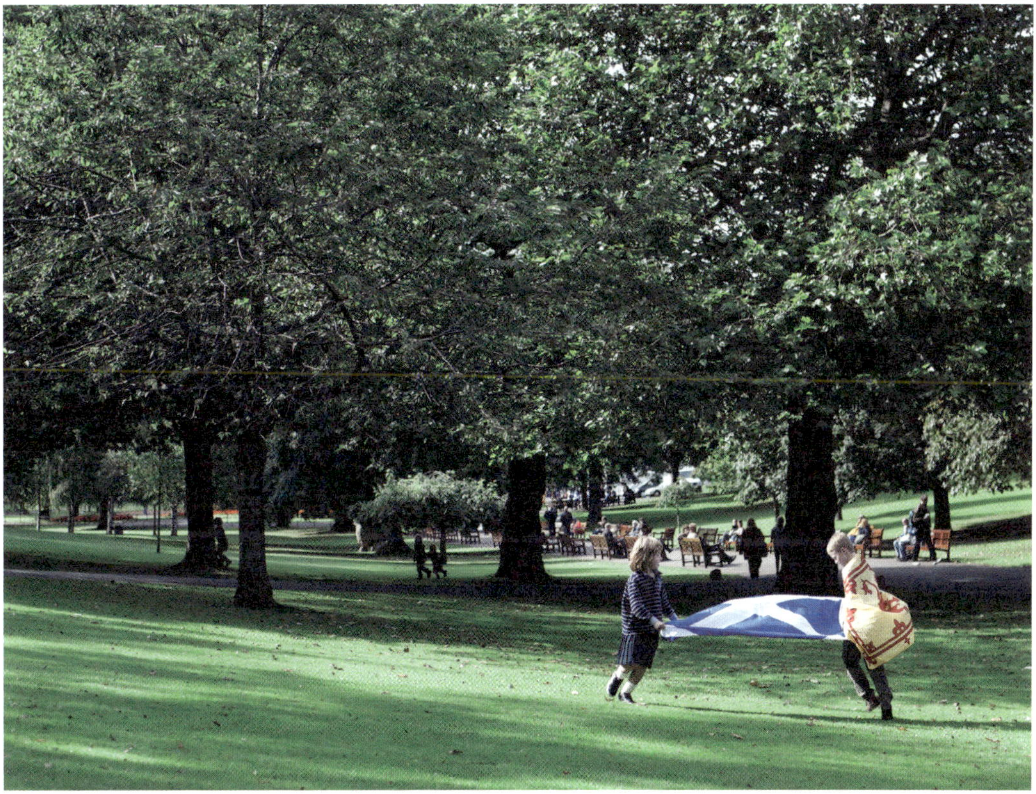

Peter McNally / Documenting Yes

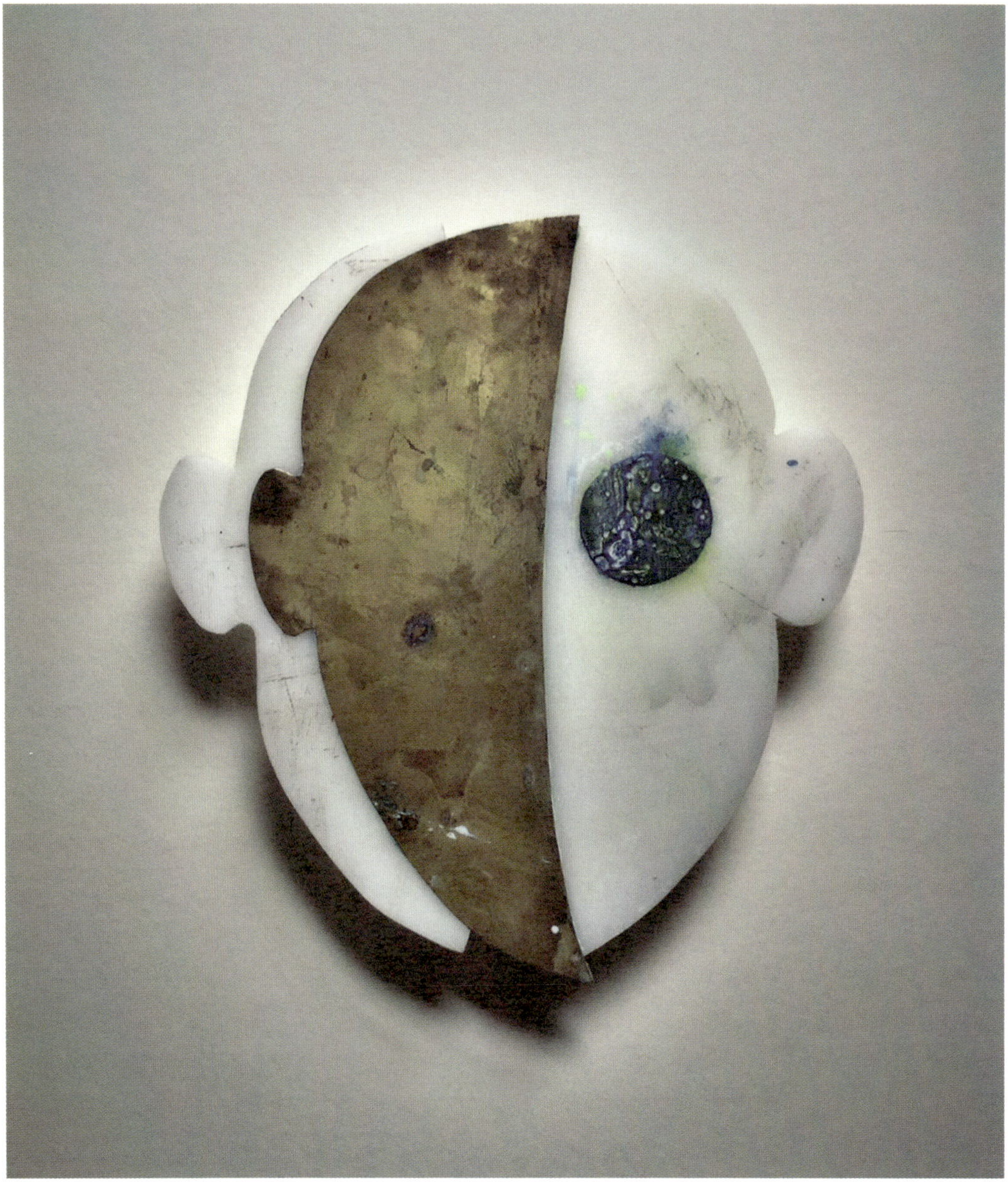

Mind
Eoghann MacColl

Indian Leaf Butterfly

Tessa Ransford

Underwings brown and sere
tapered to a stalk
folded and creased
as a dead leaf
or a prayer

Opened wings reveal
bold blue and gold
black fringed
with white rings
and strains of purple in the paler blue
luminous, surreal

Prove in flight the inside
(or the out)
the back (or front)
when all seems dead and withered
winging on

Thanks

Max Wiszniewski

Chris Silver

Susa Rae

David Carr

Elaine Smith

Paul Crawford

Willie Sullivan

Lindsay Conn

Robin McAlpine

Katie Gallogly-Swan

Benjamin Wray

Cristina Ertze

Jean Mingo

Thomas Burn

Pauline Goldsmith

With special thanks to Tessa for contributing to this book during her illness – and for being such a firm friend of Common Weal

Scott Langdon

David Whyte

Jennifer Volk

Scott Hames

Aileen McKay

Frances Rougvie

Gemma Maramis

Adam Turner

Jim Bevington

Angela Haggerty

Phil Connor

Stuart McHardy

Tommy Sheppard

Joan Docherty

Daniel James

Suzy Lickley

Tarlochan Gata-Aura

Moira Paterson

Credits

Page 13	From Sullivan, W; *The Missing Scotland:Why over a million Scots choose not to vote and what it means for our democracy*; Luath Press; Edinburgh; 2014; www.luath.co.uk
Page 17	From RIC Declaration, 2013; Radical Independence Campaign; 2013; radicalindependence.org
Page 24	From Polwart, K; *Imagination vital to telling the Yes story*; The Scotsman, Online; 17 February, 2013; www.scotsman.com
Page 31	From Bathurst, B; *Salmond and Darling squabble, but the real conversation about the Scottish referendum is elsewhere;* The Guardian, Online; 10 August 2014; www.theguardian.com
Page 33	From Bjork; Facebook; 17 September, 2014
Page 37 & 43	From *Common Weal: The Book*; Scottish Left Review Press; 2014; www.allofusfirst.org
Page 45	From Small, M; *An Independent Media for Scotland?*; Bella Caledonia, Online; 26 September, 2014; www.bellacaledonia.org.uk
Page 55	From Sillars, J: *In Place of Fear II*; Vagabond Voices; Glasgow; 2014; www.vagabondvoices.co.uk
Page 60	From Welsh, I; *Scottish Independence and British Unity*; Bella Caledonia, Online; 10 January, 2013; www.bellacaledonia.org.uk
Page 61	From Wightman, A; *Balmoral Buyout*; Bella Caledonia, Online; 19 November, 2007; www.bellacaledonia.org.uk
Page 63	From Riddoch, L; *Blossom*; Luath Press; Edinburgh; 2013. www.luath.co.uk
Page 73	From RIC Declaration 2012; Radical Independence Campaign; 2012; www.radicalindependence.org
Page 75	From Ferguson, N; *Scottish referendum: Alone, Scotland will go back to being a failed state*; The Telegraph, Online; 17 September, 2014; www.telegraph.co.uk
Page 83	From Cochrane, A; *Alex Salmond: My Part In His Downfall*; Biteback Publishing; 2014; www.bitebackpublishing.com
Page 88	From *The Common Weal book of policy proposals for the 2016 Scottish elections*, forthcoming on Common Print; www.allofusfirst.org
Page 89	From McDermid, V; *Scottish writers on the referendum – Independence day?*; The Guardian, Online; 19 July, 2014; www.theguardian.com
Page 91	From McAlpine, R; *Wipe your eyes. On your feet*; Bella Caledonia, Online; 19 September, 2014; www.bellacaledonia.org.uk
Page 98	From Boyd, C; Morrison, J; *Scottish Independence – A Feminist Response*; Word Power Books; 2014; www.word-power.co.uk
Page 101	From Smith, D; McHardy, S; *Scotland's Democracy Trail*; Luath Press; Edinburgh; 2014; www.luath.co.uk
Page 107	From Gray, A; *Work as if you live in the early days of a better nation*; Herald Scotland, Online; 5 May, 2007; www.heraldscotland.com/